UNDERGROUND CURES

The Most Urgent Health Secrets

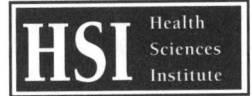

Published by Agora Health Books
Anne Kelly, Publisher
Ken Danz, Copy Editor
Martin Milner, N.D., Medical Editor

© Copyright 2000 by Agora Health Books, 819 N. Charles St., Baltimore, MD 21201. All rights reserved. No part of this book may be reproduced by any means or for any reason without the consent of the publisher. The information contained herein is obtained from sources believed to be reliable, but its accuracy cannot be guaranteed.

ISBN 1-891434-05-5

Additional orders and inquiries can be directed to the Health Sciences Institute, Members Services Department, 702 Cathederal St., Baltimore, MD 21201; tel. (800)851-7100 or(410) 223-2611, fax (410) 223-2619.

All material in this publication is provided for information only and may not be construed as medical advice or instruction. No action or inaction should be taken based solely on the contents of this publication; instead, readers should consult appropriate health professionals on any matter relating to their health and well-being. The information and opinions provided in this publication are believed to be accurate and sound, based on the best judgment available to the authors, but readers who fail to consult with appropriate health authorities assume the risk of any injuries. The publisher is not responsible for errors or omissions.

THE INFORMATION PRESENTED HERE HAS NOT BEEN EVALUATED BY THE U.S. FOOD & DRUG ADMINISTRATION. THIS PRODUCT IS NOT INTENDED TO DIAGNOSE, TREAT, CURE, OR PREVENT ANY DISEASE.

Table of Contents

Introduction

SECTION I Super Immunity for the Millenium

Chapter 1
Calcium Elenolate: Nature's Most Powerful Antibiotic — 3

Chapter 2
The Lactoferrin Miracle — 7

Chapter 3
Infopeptides: The Next Generation Immune Booster — 13

Chapter 4
Probiotics: Help for the Postantibiotic World — 17

SECTION II Cancer-free for the 21st Century

Chapter 5
Modified Citrus Pectin (MCP):
Halt the Most Lethal Process at Work — 25

Chapter 6
Glycoalkaloids: a New Non-Surgical Solution for Skin Cancer — 29

Chapter 7
PC Specs: New "Hope" for Prostate Cancer — 35

Chapter 8
Breast-Cancer Detection:
Making Breast Self-Exams Easier to Perform — 41

Chapter 9
Phytochemicals: Nature's "Super Foods" — 47

SECTION III A Stronger Heart for the Next Century

Chapter 10
Cardiocysteine: Reduce your Risk of Heart Disease — 53

Chapter 11
Freeze-Frame: 60 Seconds to a Longer Life — 59

Chapter 12
Organic Germanium: "Electrify" Your Health — 63

SECTION IV New Solutions for Auto-immune Diseases

Chapter 13
Thymic Formula Reverses Hepatitis,
Rheumatoid Arthritis and More — 69

Chapter 14
Shark Cartilage Therapy:
Help Your Body Create NEW Cartilage — 75

Chapter 15
    Nutrient Discovery Prevents and Reverses Osteoporosis   81

Chapter 16
    Formula from Ancient Asia Controls Rheumatoid Arthritis   85

Chapter 17
    Larreastat: Relief for Victims of
    Herpes and Rheumatoid Arthritis   91

SECTION V Boost Brain Power and Manage Mental Health

Chapter 18
    Phosphatidylserine...the One True Smart Pill   99

Chapter 19
    DHA: Boost Your Brainpower   103

Chapter 20
    Inositol: Nutrient Therapy for Alzheimer's
    Disease, Depression and Anxiety   105

Chapter 21
    Kava Kava: The Feel-Good
    Herb of the South Pacific   109

SECTION VI Super Sex for as Long as You Want

Chapter 22
    V-Power: Promote Your Sexual Health   115

Chapter 23
    Yam Cream for Men and Women:
    Restore Optimum Hormone Levels   121

Chapter 24
    Red Deer Antler Velvet:
    Animal-Like Results   127

SECTION VII Powerful Pain Relief Solutions

Chapter 25
    XP-100: A Gentle Alternative to Ibuprofen   135

Chapter 26
    Farabloc Blanket: Banish Pain Without Drugs   139

Chapter 27
    Migraine Formula: Relief from Migraines...Naturally   145

Guide to Sources and Availability   147

Index   153

Health Sciences Institute Membership Information   159

Introduction

The inaugural edition of *Underground Cures*, published in 1998, brought together for the first time the most urgent health discoveries from the world's most progressive health clinics and research laboratories. This year, Agora Health Books has once again partnered with Health Sciences Institute to bring you the updated edition of *Underground Cures*, which contains a hidden universe of remedies and healing possibilities you never imagined existed. The mainstream medical establishment and even many alternative medical communities have yet to discover these advanced, underground cures and urgent health breakthroughs.

This edition of *Underground Cures* is packed with 27 new chapters containing secrets for enhancing your health, extending your life, and liberating yourself from the devastating effects of many serious conditions. We've also reorganized the contents so you can quickly find the section you're looking for, whether it's breakthrough solutions for immuno-support, degenerative and autoimmune disorders and viruses, cancer, brainpower and mental health, energy, sexual health, heart health, or pain relief.

Every day, around the world, researchers and scientists are making exciting medical breakthroughs and health discoveries. Yet, you are often deprived of these healing possibilities. Your doctor may be too busy to sift through all the latest research. Or maybe he is overly influenced by the big pharmaceutical companies. Or perhaps a potentially lifesaving treatment is trapped in the tangles of government bureaucracy. The bottom line is this...for one reason or another, you are not getting the health information you need when you need it.

In 1996, a small, private group of conventionally and holistically trained doctors formed a network through which they could rapidly exchange news of the latest, most innovative cures and overcome bureaucratic blocks and delays.

This network is the Health Sciences Institute, dedicated to uncovering and researching the most urgent advances in modern underground medicine, like those in this book. The hard work and commitment of these "underground" health pioneers brings these cures to light...so that you can use them today.

The Health Sciences Institute now has over 75,000 members worldwide. As it grows in international reputation, more and more laboratories and scientists send news of their research directly to the institute. The editors at HSI research the truly revolutionary breakthroughs for safety, efficacy, and availability.

Every day, stacks of letters arrive from people whose lives were changed by a breakthrough they learned of through the HSI network. The institute maintains a file of members who have overcome such diseases as arthritis, prostate disorders, fatigue, and depression...of members who, although they had nearly given up hope, experienced dramatic recoveries when they tried a remedy they read about in an HSI publication. Please turn to page 159 to find out how you can receive regular news of the latest medical breakthroughs by becoming a member of the Health Sciences Institute.

SECTION I
Super Immunity for the Millenium

In today's world, we are constantly assaulted by a growing number of environmental and biological threats to our health. There's simply no way to avoid the drug-resistant bacteria, industrial chemicals, and nutrient-depleted foods that depress our natural immune responses and leave us vulnerable. The best defense? To develop disease resistance at the cellular level—in short, to achieve superimmunity.

In this section, you'll learn about a new generation of natural immune-system boosters that may provide the most effective health insurance you can buy. Read on to learn how you can resist and overcome the most serious health threats of our age.

1

Calcium Elenolate: Nature's Most Powerful Antibiotic

Tomorrow's #1 Threat to Your Health Is Here Today

You may not believe it now, but infectious "smart bugs" are going to be the No. 1 threat to your health. In the past 15 years, death by infectious disease has already gone from being the fifth-leading killer in the United States to being the third-leading one!

And now, nine disease-causing bugs—bugs we thought we'd beaten long ago—have returned, stronger than the original strains...bringing a plague of dangerous and even deadly illnesses, including blood poisoning, tuberculosis, meningitis, pneumonia, sinusitis, gonorrhea, and bacteremia.

Once, doctors could destroy these bacteria with powerful drugs. That was back in the golden age of antibiotics. Today, it doesn't matter how quickly we invent drugs to kill them. Faster than we can create new antibiotics in our laboratories, deadly bacteria are developing resistance to the potent but limited drugs. There is one way, however, to stop these superbugs. We can outsmart them, using the tremendous protective power of nature.

Nature's most promising antibiotic, antiviral, and antifungal agent is a compound derived from the olive leaf, called calcium elenolate. As the number of drug-resistant superbugs continues to increase, so will the urgent need for olive-leaf extract.

This plant extract not only helps your body battle the dangerous bugs that cause infectious disease but also detoxifies your entire system, enhances your energy, improves your circulation, activates key components of your immune system, and has beneficial effects on cholesterol and blood-sugar levels.

The history of calcium elenolate

Treatments made from the olive-leaf extract have been around for at least 150 years, with records dating back to 1827, when it was used as a treatment for malaria—with no side effects other than those produced by the ethanol wine used in these special ethanolic preparations. In 1906, the olive-leaf extract was reportedly far superior to quinine for the treatment of malaria, but quinine, because it was easier to administer, became the treatment of choice.

In 1957, the active ingredient of olive-leaf extract, oleuropein, was isolated and studied as a treatment for high blood pressure and other types of heart disease, again with no mention of toxic or other side effects.

From 1970 to the present, a hydrolyzed form of oleuropein has been tested and found effective against dozens of different viruses and many strains of bacteria. None of these experiments noted any toxicity.

Now in tablet form, olive-leaf extract is making a comeback. From Mexico we have reports describing dramatic malaria remissions, but the therapeutic potential of the olive leaf is much more far-reaching. It's been proven to work in a number of specific ways:

- It stunts the growth of viruses or bacteria by interfering with certain amino-acid production processes necessary for those pathogens to grow.
- It inhibits the spread of the pathogen by preventing shedding, budding, or assembly at the cell membrane (i.e., it inactivates the virus or bacterium).
- It can enter your infected cells and shut down viral replication processes.
- In the case of retroviruses, such as HIV, it neutralizes the production of enzymes that are essential for a retrovirus to alter the RNA of a healthy cell.
- It directly stimulates phagocytosis—your immune system's ability to "eat" foreign microorganisms that don't belong in your body.

Clearly, this substance is highly complex—much more so than synthetic antibiotics—and this complexity is one of the keys to its success.

The importance of natural antibiotics in a dangerous age of infectious diseases

Independent research has shown that olive-leaf extract can be used as an adjunct treatment for influenza, meningitis, the Epstein-Barr virus (EBV), encephalitis, the common cold, herpes I and II, HHV-6, HHV-7, shingles, HTLV-I, HTLV-II, HIV/ARC/AIDS, CFIDS, CMV, hepatitis B, pneumonia, sinusitis, tuberculosis, gonorrhea, malaria, bacteremia, urinary-tract infections, severe diarrhea, blood poisoning, and surgical infections.

Because it's a natural substance, olive-leaf extract has a much wider range of actions than man-made antibiotics. It contains a maze of chemicals—harmless to us—that lie in wait for invading bacteria. In this way, olive-leaf extract is very much like garlic, the traditional herbal cure-all. Garlic contains 17 amino acids, and 33 sulfur compounds, plus copper, germanium, selenium, zinc, calcium, iron, potassium, magnesium, and vitamins A, B-1, and C-2. As you can imagine, it is much more difficult for an invading bacterium to develop resistance in the face of such a complex mixture of active chemicals.

Plant medicines like olive-leaf extract offer a great deal of promise for the future treatment of infectious diseases. According to experts at the Centers for Disease Control in Atlanta, medicine must continue to probe natural resources if it is to provide effective health care for all. Nature has evolved germ killers far more potent than any that laboratory scientists can invent. The olive-leaf extract is one of these germ killers.

The safety factor

In 1970, the Upjohn Pharmaceutical Company conducted and published a safety study on the use of olive-leaf extract in lab animals. An extrapolation of Upjohn's figures reveals that even at doses several hundred times the recommended amount, no toxic or other adverse side effects are likely to appear.

Bonus heart-health benefits of this special olive-leaf compound

The Mediterranean diet, rich in vegetables, fruits, grains, and olive oil, has recently been linked to a low incidence of heart disease. According to many studies, the olive-leaf compound has been found to serve as a vasodilator (it opens up your blood vessels), to prevent LDL oxidation (which causes hardened arteries), and even to help with diabetes and high blood pressure.

It thoroughly cleanses and detoxifies your system. In fact, the manufacturers of olive-leaf-extract supplements warn that you may experience significant detoxification symptoms. These symptoms—which can vary from stomach rumblings and other digestive disorders to mild headaches—are positive signs that the supplement is "at work." You can lessen these side effects, however, with a program of vitamin C supplementation, taken to bowel tolerance, and/or a probiotic formula to ensure strong, beneficial microflora in your bowel.

Generally, the recommended amount of olive-leaf extract is one or two 500-milligram tablets daily. After about two weeks, you can increase the amount to six or eight capsules daily. When you begin to feel better, reduce the amount to one or two capsules daily.

Please turn to the "Guide to Sources and Availability" on page 147 for information on obtaining olive-leaf extract (calcium elenolate).

2

LACTOFERRIN:
THE HEALING MYSTERY OF MOTHERS' MILK

History may reveal the discovery of lactoferrin to be among the most important medical advancements of the 20th century. This potent, natural immune booster has been reported to hinder tumor growth and metastasis, relieve the suffering of AIDS-related complexes, and protect the immunologically vulnerable from deadly viruses and bacterial infections. In healthy individuals, it can mean near-total immunity from colds, influenza, microbial parasites, and infectious bacteria. Its healing powers appear to be unrivaled. And yet, lactoferrin remains largely unknown and poorly understood, even in the alternative medical community.

What is lactoferrin and where does it come from?

Lactoferrin is an immune chemical produced by the body as part of its shield against infection. In a healthy individual, it's found in secretions like tears, perspiration, the lining of the intestinal tract, and the mucous membranes that line the nose, ears, throat, and urinary tract—in short, any place that is especially vulnerable to infection.

But by far the highest concentrations of lactoferrin are found in a substance called colostrum (or "first milk"), produced by a new mother in the first few hours after she gives birth. For the newborn, lactoferrin provides crucial immune-system stimulation, helping the new baby to survive in its new germ-laden environment outside the womb.

Recently, scientists have discovered that using lactoferrin in the form of a nutritional supplement can significantly boost the immune system and greatly enhance the body's ability to withstand and recover from infection and other illness. Lactoferrin supplements are produced using bovine colostrum. The process used to create the commercial preparation leaves the lactoferrin protein intact and chemically unaltered. (For those who are allergic to milk or lactose-intolerant, please note that the milk sugars responsible for lactose intolerance and the proteins responsible for cow's-milk allergies are largely absent in bovine colostrum. Except in the case of extreme sensitivity, lactoferrin usually presents no problems for those with milk sensitivities.)

Have you noticed?
The "common" cold is becoming a thing of the past

It used to be that you could expect to get one or two colds a season—a few days of sinus congestion, maybe a scratchy throat. Nowadays, it's not uncommon to suffer half a dozen major viral infections a year. Family physicians report the increasing prevalence of "super cold" viruses—colds that wipe you out for two weeks or more with bone-wearying fatigue, debilitating throat and sinus pain, and a nagging cough that drags on for weeks or even develops into bronchitis.

For anyone who is immune-impaired for any reason—recovering from surgery or cancer therapy, for example, the stakes are much higher: Even one bad cold can lead to hospitalization, or even become life-threatening.

And then there's the flu. Even flu shots can't adequately protect you. New and increasingly dangerous strains of the flu appear each year, circling the globe with astonishing speed.

Your only defense is a strong immune system

You can't avoid exposure to these infections, but you can help ensure that your immune system is strong enough to knock the bugs out before they take hold in your body. Research indicates that lactoferrin supplementation may be your key to developing this kind of superimmunity. Lactoferrin increases both the number and the activity of at least half-dozen different types of specific immune cells that help your body fight infection.

By taking supplemental lactoferrin daily (100 to 300 mg) as a preventive regimen, you're more likely to stay well while co-workers and acquaintances pass around the same cold or flu. When you sense that you might be "coming down with something," you can increase the amount (to 500 mg) in order to increase the level of protection.

Lactoferrin's actions extend far beyond the "cold and flu" season. Research has documented a long list of remarkable benefits, especially against retroviruses and malignancies. Lactoferrin can inhibit the growth of both tumors and metastasis, and scientists studying it report that it may be one of the best protective regimens against tumor formation and excessive cell proliferation available.

How does lactoferrin work?

Lactoferrin is a type of cytokine—an immune chemical that helps coordinate the body's cellular immune response, defending against invaders like bacteria and viruses. In particular, it functions as a type of border guard: It patrols the tissues at the openings of the body-nose, eyes, and mouth, as well as cuts or abrasions in the skin-for pathogens that can harm you. In the event of an invasion of microbes, your body increases production of lactoferrin, which is directly toxic to bacteria, yeast, and molds.

The most distinguishing characteristic of lactoferrin is its ability to bind to iron in the blood, denying tumor cells, bacteria, and viruses the iron they need to survive and multiply. But as researchers continue to test lactoferrin against various disease processes, several more important functions have been revealed. Lactoferrin also has been documented to:

- enhance natural "killer-cell" activity (which targets specific types of tumors and virus-infected cells)
- activate neutrophil cells (which surround and digest foreign bodies)
- prevent bacterial overgrowth in the gut, preventing dysbiosys
- prevent viruses (including those that cause AIDS, herpes, heart disease, and some types of cancer) from penetrating into your healthy cells
- inhibit tumor growth and metastasis
- reduce inflammation—which can reduce pain and increase mobility
- inhibit Candida albicans and other Candida strains
- inhibit free-radical production—fighting the aging effects of cellular oxidation
- function as an inhibitor of mammary cell growth—which means it may hold promise for prevention or treatment of breast cancer
- play a role in lessening ocular disturbances—which means it may help with vision problems
- act as a potent antimicrobial agent against Candida albicans

Studies suggest that with lactoferrin, "more is better." The more lactoferrin that is present in the body, the more effectively it performs its many immune-stimulating functions. There appears to be no toxic dosage—which is not surprising when you consider that high concentrations of lactoferrin are well tolerated by newborn infants.

Widely used to support recovery from cancer

Numerous studies have documented the benefits of lactoferrin against many types of cancer, including leukemia, Hodgkin's disease, and cancers involving the colon, breast, and lung.

Many holistic practitioners use it to achieve great effects by combining it with other immune-enhancing natural cancer therapies. In one widely reported case, a patient who had not been responding particularly well to a program of natural cancer therapies suddenly showed almost miraculous improvement when lactoferrin was added to her regime. This seemingly "hopeless" case was transformed into a remarkable recovery.

Other case histories indicate that the negative effects of conventional cancer treatments like chemotherapy and radiation are drastically reduced or eliminated with supplemental lactoferrin. (The amounts of lactoferrin used in these reported cases ranges from 500 to 1,500 mg per day.) Again, it should be noted that lactoferrin appears to be perfectly safe, even in high amounts.

Lactoferrin in stroke recovery

A member of the HSI network had suffered three strokes by the age of 68.

After two days of lactoferrin supplementation, she reports, "I was in the house cooking, doing everything I'd always done. I'm still taking my medication for my heart attack, but I feel great! I have a lot of energy.

"Before, I couldn't speak plainly because of the stroke, but I can talk now! My speech has come back. Also, I hadn't been able to drive because my eyesight was so bad, but after a short time on the lactoferrin, I can drive again!"

Lactoferrin appears to have a profound effect on degenerative (as opposed to infectious) disease. Although we can't say yet exactly how, it's very possible that lactoferrin's antioxidant action plays a key role. As you know, free radicals oxidize the LDL (bad) cholesterol, which causes arteries to harden and circulation to suffer.

Hope for autistic and brain-damaged children

Lactoferrin may even hold significant hope for children with autism or brain injuries. Nutritional biochemist Patricia Kane of Millville, New Jersey, has begun working with autistic and brain-injured children and has witnessed surprising results with the administration of lactoferrin.

Although autism is a brain dysfunction, Dr. Kane points out that, because of the involvement of the entire body, improvement can only come about by embracing all the systemic interactions—a holistic approach. The use of lactoferrin represents significant progress toward this goal. Protection against the cryptosporidium parasites Cryptosporidium parasites cause acute diarrhea in people with strong, healthy immune systems but can be life-threatening in those who are immune compromised. Studies published in *Infection & Immunity* (no. 61, 1993, pp. 4079) have shown that colostrum is able to ameliorate or completely eliminate the clinical symptoms of those suffering from cryptosporidiosis.

Stops lethal and debilitating viruses—including HIV and herpes—from replicating

Lactoferrin appears to be able to interfere with the replication of certain viruses, including some herpes viruses. These viruses have been linked to heart disease, inflammatory bowel disease, shingles, and chronic fatigue. Lactoferrin's antiviral properties have been proven effective against HIV. (In fact, one of the first big breakthroughs in lactoferrin research occurred six years ago when a medical journal reported its success in helping AIDS patients reverse the potentially life-threatening condition of chronic diarrhea.)

Lactoferrin—a healing revolution

When you look at the number of very different immune-enhancing functions that lactoferrin performs, it's easy to wonder: Is there any health condition that lactoferrin won't help? And the truth is that doctors and healers are discovering new uses for lactoferrin almost as quickly as they can test them. Even more importantly, you now have direct access to this revolutionary new tool for immune system activation. For information on purchasing lactoferrin, see the "Guide to Sources and Availability" on page 149.

Actions:
- Activates DNA that launches the immune response
- Activates neutrophil cells that surround and digest foreign bodies
- Binds with iron in the blood
- Acts as an antioxidant
- Acts as an anti-inflammatory

Benefits:
- Enhances natural killer (NK cell) activity that targets specific types of tumors and virus-infected cells
- Nutritionally deprives cancer cells and bacteria of the iron they need for metabolism and proliferation
- Prevents bacterial overgrowth in the gut, preventing dysbiosis
- Inhibits free-radical production
- Reduces inflammation, which can reduce pain and increase mobility

References
"Bovine Lactoferrin and Lactoferricin inhibit tumor metastasis in mice," *Jpn. J. Cancer Res.* vol. 88, pp. 184-190, 1997.

"Human lactoferrin inhibits growth of solid tumors and metastases in mice," *Cancer Research*, vol. 54, no. 9, pp. 2310-2, 1994.

"Modulation of natural killer and lymphokine-activated killer cell cytotoxicity by lactoferrin," *J. Leukocyte Biology*, vol. 51, pp. 343-349, 1992.

"Influence of lactoferrin on the function of human polymorphonuclear leukocytes and monocytes," *J. Leukocyte Biology*, vol. 49, pp. 427-433, 1991.

"Lactoferrin inhibits bacterial translocation in mice fed bovine milk," *Applied and Environmental Microbiology*, vol. 61, no. 11, pp. 4131-4134, 1995.

"Inhibition with Lactoferrin of in vitro infection with HHV," *Jpn. J. of Medical Science and Biology*, vol. 472, pp. 735, 1994.

"The Role of Lactoferrin as an anti-inflammatory molecule," *Advances in Experimental Medicine and Biology*, vol. 357, pp. 143-156, 1994.

"Killing of Candida Albicans by Lactoferricin B," *Medical Microbiology and Immunology*, vol. 182, no. 2, pp. 97-105, 1993.

3

INFOPEPTIDES:
THE NEXT GENERATION IMMUNE BOOSTER

The Health Sciences Institute has been tracking the progress of a truly amazing natural product that has successfully treated everything from acute viral attacks to serious, chronic, and even life-threatening disorders. But until recently, this substance was available only to the small number of physicians involved in or aware of the research. We can finally share news of the healing potential of infopeptides, because an infopeptide product is now available to you.

On the basis of research done thus far, infopeptides have the potential to revolutionize at least three major areas of treatment:

(1) immune dysfunctions (from minor to major, including AIDS)
(2) childhood diarrhea
(3) myalgias and muscle pains, including arthritis and fibromyalgia

Recently, physicians at one of the most important and successful cancer centers in the world, Klinik St. George in Bad Aibling, Germany, became aware of this research. They are so impressed that they are using this product, along with lactoferrin (see Chapter 2) to treat 100 cancer patients.

Biochemical research finds a previously unknown compound in colostrum

Infopeptides are a type of peptide found in milk and colostrum (the mother's "first milk") and were not previously known to exist. They are fundamentally different from whole colostrum and from lactoferrin because they appear to have no direct antiviral or antibacterial properties of their own. They do, however, contain chemically coded instructions that appear to be vitally important to a properly regulated immune system.

Infopeptides, however, are not found naturally in breast milk. The longer peptide chains have to be broken down into shorter segments in order to work. This appears to happen *naturally* in the process of sucking milk from the breast—probably a result of a combination of physical manipulation and enzymes in the mouth of the newborn. Once they are activated in this way, infopeptides have an impressive ability to trigger powerful antiviral, antibacterial, and antiprotozoal immune functions. In that sense, their action is more hormone like than nutrientlike. But they seem to be self-regulating in a way that artificial hormones are not. As noted by Staroscik, et al. in *Molecular Immunology* (vol. 210, no. 120, pp. 1277-82):

A small-chain polyprotein-rich peptide in colostrum...has the same ability to regulate the activity of the immune system as the hormones of the thymus gland do. It activates an underactive immune system, helping it move into action against disease-causing organisms. It also suppresses an overactive immune system, such as is often seen in the autoimmune diseases.

It also appears to act on T cell precursors to produce helper T cells and suppressor T cells. The effect is similar to that of thymus hormones.

(Note: This country's most widely prescribed drug—synthetic estrogen—reduces the function of the thymus.)

Infopeptides are unique because of their ability to control both underactive and overactive immune systems (*Archives of Immunology & Therapeutic Experiments*, vol. 41, nos. 5-6, pp. 275-9, 1993). Research has linked these polypeptides to widespread biological actions that alleviate inflammation, nervous disorders, and even sleep patterns (*Trends in Neuroscience*, vol. 18, no. 3, pp. 130-6, 1995).

Another exciting aspect of the infopeptide mode of action is that it is not dose-dependent. That is, once a very small amount of an infopeptide is consumed, an increased dose does nothing more.

Help for arthritis, fibromyalgia, AIDS, and more

"Cytolog" is the name given to infopeptide products developed by a company that has been studying infopeptides since 1992. In a small-scale study, 82 percent of rheumatoid-arthritis patients experienced "good or very good" results within two to six weeks with the use of Cytolog. Subjects with osteoarthritis all reported "good or very good" responses; one patient is in complete remission. All of the patients had been taking at least one drug, and many of them had been taking up to four drugs—all to no avail.

The participants had been suffering from six to 20 years.

Cytolog helped to fight acute (and potentially lethal) diarrhea in children in Guatemala. Worldwide, between 5 and 10 million children die every year from diarrhea...making the implications of this research profound.

In another, as-yet-unpublished study, this one in Baltimore, AIDS patients showed a 50 percent reduction in symptoms in a short period of time with just 5 to 10 milliliters of Cytolog per day.

It will be months or even years before these findings appear in major medical journals, but because they are so significant, we are trying to get the word out as quickly as possible.

Doctors report incredible recoveries

Jeff Anderson, M.D., of Corte Madera, California, described his own experience with Cytolog after he contracted viral myalgic meningoencephalitis (a brain inflammation). He used two 5-milliliter doses per day for a week and found the results nothing short of amazing. He encountered rapid relief of inflammatory-connective-tissue pain (particularly myalgic pain and stiffness, as well as headache) within two or three minutes.

Dr. Arnold Takemoto, from Scottsdale, Arizona, stated that he thought the reports on Cytolog "too good to be true" when he first tested it clinically. He has been working with more than 500 active patients with medical problems that baffle traditional allopathic medicine. Dr. Takemoto's specialties are chronic fatigue immune-deficiency syndrome and fibromyalgia (two of the fastest-growing diseases among women), along with specialized consultation on referred patients who have stage-4 cancer. Takemoto reports that his patients are experiencing incredible results with Cytolog.

Shingles, digestive problems, joint pain: All show dramatic improvement

Teresa E. Quinlin, M.D., of Winchester, Ohio, has seen dramatic improvement in acute viral illnesses, including shingles. Gastritis and other digestive problems have also been quickly resolved. One woman suffering from polymyalgia rheumatica (a painful disease of the collagen tissue) had a 90 percent reduction in joint and muscle pain. Dr. Quinlin hopes to see a total remission in this case.

Are cows good enough?

Is the bovine source just as good as the human derivation? The answer is probably yes. Bovine colostrum and lactoferrin are close but not precise matches to human counterparts. Certain infopeptides from cows, however, are believed to be 100 percent identical to those found in human milk.

For those who are lactose intolerant, it's also important to recognize that milk sugars responsible for lactose intolerance and the proteins responsible for cow's-milk allergies are largely absent in colostrum.

Considering the small doses needed for effectiveness and the very small concentration of lactose remaining, the use of colostrum products should be of no concern to those with milk sensitivities.

Cytolog appears to be safe and well-tolerated when taken under a variety of circumstances and over extended periods of time. The benefits do not diminish but tend to increase over time. In fact, those who take Cytolog for three months or more relate that the benefits persist indefinitely even after they stop taking it.

We predict that you'll be hearing much more about infopeptides in the very near future. See the "Guide to Sources and Availability" on page 149.

Actions:
- Regulates the activity of the immune system
- Acts on T-cell precursors to produce helper T-cells and suppressor T-cells
- Triggers antiviral, antibacterial, and antiprotozoal functions

Benefits:
- Activates an underactive immune system, helping it fight disease-causing organisms
- Suppresses an overactive immune system, which is often seen in autoimmune diseases
- Alleviates inflammation
- Relieves myalgic pain and stiffness

4

PROBIOTICS:
HELP FOR THE POSTANTIBIOTIC AGE

During World War II, a new wonder drug emerged: It was penicillin, the very first antibiotic. Today, "antibiotic" is a household word. It literally means "destructive of life," and the term is generally applied to substances that can kill or inhibit the growth of undesirable microorganisms. Now, of course, we know the sad truth: Antibiotics also annihilate beneficial microorganisms.

Probiotics are food supplements that encourage the growth and proliferation of the microorganisms that you want to have inside your body.

("Probiotic" means "promoting life.") Probiotic supplements, such as acidophilus, are now common, and for good reason. Average adults have several thousand billion bacteria in their digestive tracts—adding up to about 4 pounds of living material. Approximately 400 different species are represented. This complex mass of life forms, an entire ecosystem in miniature, is so vital to health that it's often thought of as an organ in its own right.

Up until now, probiotic supplementation has been largely an act of faith. These bacteria are exquisitely sensitive to light, air, temperature, and pH balance. In a typical probiotic supplement, whatever live organisms survive the manufacturing process, shipping, and storage are destroyed by digestive juices in your stomach before they reach their target.

In addition, it is difficult to effectively isolate the desired organisms from competing strains. The cultures in which the probiotic bacteria are grown are easily contaminated with other, undesirable strains of bacteria, which then hitch a ride into your system.

But now, a significant advance in probiotic technology lays these issues to rest. A newly identified strain of lactobacillus demonstrates unprecedented potency in humans, as well as unparalleled stability and shelf life. After reviewing scores of scientific studies, clinical trials, and product assays, we're convinced that this new substance provides—by far—the best probiotic support available.

You have billions of bacteria in your gut—if you're lucky

In a healthy individual, beneficial bacteria inhabit the digestive tract in massive numbers, crowding out harmful bacteria, aiding digestion, and supporting the body's immune function. This healthy "gut flora" produces valuable nutrients (including certain B vitamins and short-chain fatty acids), digestive enzymes like lactase, and immune chemicals that fight harmful bacteria and even cancer cells.

But this critical ecosystem is fragile and easily disturbed. Antibiotic therapy can completely kill off the beneficial bacteria in the gut along with the intended target.

Steroid drugs like cortisone and prednisone, as well as birth-control pills, can severely upset your gut flora, as can chemotherapeutic drugs. In addition, poor nutrition or digestion can impair the efficiency of intestinal bacteria, as can stress, trauma, surgery, or parasitic infestation. When the number or activity level of your good bacteria drops too low, it opens the door for harmful bacteria to proliferate—and disease to develop.

Perhaps the most commonly known example is candidiasis, in which Candida bacteria multiply out of control, causing a widespread systemic breakdown.

Other pernicious diseases have been linked to intestinal overgrowth of specific bacteria as well. For example, rheumatoid arthritis has been associated with Proteus bacteria and ankylosing spondylitis with the Klebsiella strain.[1]

Even more commonly, intestinal imbalance (or dysbiosis) can cause damage to the protective tissue that lines the intestines, leading to "leaky gut syndrome." Left untreated, leaky gut syndrome can trigger a vicious cycle of associated symptoms and systemic dysfunctions.

If you can't beat 'em...eat 'em

By introducing good bacteria in sufficient numbers, it is possible to "recolonize" the digestive tract, crowding out bad bacteria with beneficial ones. While eating cultured products like yogurt and kefir can help maintain good intestinal flora, these foods cannot provide organisms in the vast numbers required to correct an imbalance. For this, you need a high-potency probiotic nutritional supplement.

Your options just got a whole lot better

Over 10 years ago, scientists Sherwood Gorbach and Barry Goldin set out to find a strain of bacteria that could maximize the beneficial effects of probiotic supplementation. They were searching for a strain that would satisfy four basic criteria:

(1) They wanted to find a strain of lactobacillus that was native to the human digestive tract, making it more likely to flourish and proliferate in that specific environment.

(2) The bacteria had to be capable of attaching to the gut lining and reliably reproducing (or colonizing), in order to provide long-term benefits.

(3) It had to be resistant to acid and bile, able to survive the human digestive process and thus arrive in the intestines intact.

(4) It had to be perfectly safe and produce demonstrable health benefits.

For example, the bacteria commonly found in yogurt, Lactobacillus bulgaricus, is not native to human intestinal ecology. It is not designed to survive the extreme acidity of the stomach during digestion and, once in the intestines, does not efficiently attach to intestinal tissue. As a result, its benefits are relatively short-lived.

In 1985, Gorbach and Goldin discovered a previously unidentified strain of Lactobacillus bacteria that met all criteria—in fact, the subsequent research far exceeded their expectations. The new strain was named Lactobacillus G.G., after the names of its discoverers. In the intervening years, an unprecedented amount of research has been done on Lactobacillus G.G. (or LGG), documenting an astonishing range of potent beneficial actions:

- **Cancer prevention:** LGG interferes with the initiation and promotion of intestinal tumors in animal studies. Interestingly, the protective effect has been most pronounced among animals fed a high-fat diet.2 In humans, it has been shown to induce the production of immune chemicals that are the body's natural defense against cancer, such as human tumor necrosis factor, interleukin-6 and interleukin-10.3.

- **Prevention and treatment of leaky gut syndrome:** LCC helps maintain the integrity of the intestinal walls, preventing toxins from seeping through the intestines into the bloodstream and reducing intestinal inflammation. It also has been shown to reverse existing cases of increased intestinal permeability.

- **Treatment of candidiasis:** By decreasing the number of Candida in the digestive tract, LGG can both treat and prevent systemic Candida overgrowth. It has also been found that LGG stimulates the body's immune response against the Candida infection.

- **Healing of Crohn's disease:** Oral administration of LGG dramatically strengthens the gut-specific immune response in patients with Crohn's disease, as well as those with juvenile chronic arthritis (both of these being chronic inflammatory diseases associated with impaired intestinal integrity).
- **Protection against food-borne carcinogens:** Aflatoxins, toxic substances produced by molds that commonly contaminate foods—especially peanuts—are extremely harmful to the liver, causing hepatitis or even cancer. LGG has been shown to bind to and detoxify these food-borne carcinogens.
- **Treatment of virtually all types of diarrhea.** Extensive research in developing countries demonstrates the ability of LGG to treat or prevent dangerous forms of childhood diarrhea, including rotavirus as well as bacterial and relapsing diarrhea. It is also effective against traveler's diarrhea, antibiotic-associated diarrhea, and colitis, in both children and adults.

In scores of other studies, LGG has been demonstrated to increase antibody response and gut-related immune functions, protect against salmonella and clostridium, repair alcohol-related liver damage, and suppress adverse reactions in those sensitive to milk.

Recognizing the unequaled benefits of LGG, a leading nutritional-supplement manufacturer has spent the last year developing manufacturing and packaging technology that would allow mass production and distribution of this potent new strain without compromising its viability or potency.

High technology finds a solution

Having perfected a unique air- and moisture-proof packaging method, this manufacturer has produced an exceptionally potent and stable LGG supplement for the consumer market called Culturelle. Extensive testing has been done on the product to determine its shelf life under various conditions.

When refrigerated, Culturelle is guaranteed to provide an astonishing 20 billion live microorganisms per capsule, even after six months of storage. It has also been shown to be completely free of competing strains or pathogenic contamination.

The suggested dosage for ongoing probiotic support is one capsule per day. Because of the extreme potency of this product, this maintenance dosage is also frequently sufficient to resolve acute symptoms. If after two weeks you do not experience relief of your symptoms, you can increase the dosage to two capsules for a period of two or three weeks and then reduce to one capsule daily. In extremely sensitive individuals, even one capsule a day may be too potent, causing temporary diarrhea. In this case, simply break the capsules in half. See the "Guide to Sources and Availability" on page 151 for the source of Culturelle.

Actions:
- Stimulates the body's immune response
- Produces important digestive enzymes, especially lactic acid
- Produces vitamins and other trace nutrients
- Binds to and detoxifies food-borne carcinogens

Benefits:
- Maintains a healthy antibacterial and antifungal environment in the intestines
- Interferes with the initiation and promotion of intestinal tumors
- Helps maintain the integrity of the intestinal walls, preventing toxins from seeping through the intestines into the bloodstream and reducing intestinal inflammation
- Decreases the number of Candida in the digestive tract

SECTION II
Cancer-free for the 21st century

Cancer: one of the most feared diagnoses in medicine today and, unfortunately, one of the most common. Every day 3,014 Americans hear the words, "You have cancer." The good news is that the majority of them will survive it. In fact, at this moment, there are 10 million cancer survivors in this country alone. Although cancer still ends far too many lives prematurely, the death rates from some important cancers are falling. With better and earlier detection, as well as a wide range of conventional and alternative treatments, cancer is a treatable disease. More importantly, it is a preventable one.

In this section are the results of late-breaking research that confirms the roles of nutrition and natural immune-supporting substances in reducing your chances of developing this dreaded disease. You'll find chapters on phytochemicals, glycoalkaloids, breast-cancer detection, Chinese herbs for prostate cancer, and modified citrus pectin. Lactoferrin is also an important adjunct therapy for cancer: HSI research shows its promise as a supplement to traditional therapy. Read about lactoferrin in the immuno-support section of this book on page 7.

5

MODIFIED CITRUS PECTIN:
HALT THE MOST LETHAL PROCESS ON EARTH

Metastasis has been referred to as the most lethal process on earth. If it happens in your body, most doctors will consider you a grim case, at best, because metastasis refers to the spread of tumor cells from their point of origin (for example, the breast) to other organs in your body (for example, to the lymph nodes). Rarely do cancer patients die before their cancer has begun to reach out to other body parts (or metastasize). Once cancer has begun to disperse, however, it's no easy task to stop it.

Traditional weapons against metastasis—surgery, radiation, and chemotherapy (the slash, burn, and poison paradigm)—are generally considered "hit or miss." For some cancers, they may work fairly well, but even doctors who use standard treatments admit it's very difficult to target these therapies effectively. In actuality, surgery itself may cause the cancer to spread if the process hasn't already started. Radiation and chemotherapy, meant to kill wandering cancer cells, are not discriminating and kill healthy cells in the process.

The side effects of these essentially unproven treatments can include nausea, weight loss, depression, and even a critically weakened immune system. But do they work?

The truth is that despite billions of dollars spent, death rates for the major killers—lung, breast, and colon cancers—have remained essentially the same or have increased since the turn of the century. According to the U.S. National Cancer Institute, five-year relative survival rates for cancer have barely budged in the past 20 years.

But finally, scientists are beginning to find answers to important questions about the mechanisms of cancer activity, including metastasis. Research has revealed that cancer cells require special connections with normal cells in order to establish new tumor-cell colonies in other areas of the body. Various stages of this process are mediated by cell-surface components, such as carbohydrate-binding proteins.

Researchers have discovered that modified citrus pectin (MCP), which is rich in certain simple sugars, acts as an "antiadhesive agent" to prevent the cell interactions necessary for the transport and growth of tumor cells to secondary sites in the body.

Simply put, MCP targets compounds in your body that help tumor cells grow and spread. It is the first nontoxic therapy that naturally and specifically interferes with metastasis, one of the most lethal processes on earth.

Research results are pouring in
Prostate cancer

In a recent experiment at the University of Michigan Medical Center, rats were injected with a million prostate-tumor cells. Normally, metastasis would occur 10 to 12 days after injection, and the rats would die 13 to 15 days after the cancer had affected the lungs and lymph nodes.

In this study, the experimental animals received varying concentrations of modified citrus pectin in their drinking water. Some were given no MCP, some received 0.1 percent MCP, and some received 1.0 percent MCP.

There was a significant reduction in lung cancer in the animals given MCP in their drinking water for 30 days. While 15 of 16 receiving no MCP developed lung cancer in that time period, only half of those receiving 0.1 percent MCP developed lung metastases. And only one of the rats receiving the 1.0 percent MCP solution developed lung metastasis.

Lymph-node metastasis was also significantly reduced. Whereas 55 percent of the control animals developed lymph-node disease, only 13 percent of those treated with modified citrus pectin did. No toxicity was reported in any of the animals.

And the truly promising—and fascinating—news is this: The cancer-causing compound that MCP destroys in rat prostate-cancer cells (galectin-3) is also present in human tissues, including human prostate tumors! In other words, MCP may prove to work exactly the same way in human male prostate tumors as it does in rat prostate tumors.

Skin cancer

Skin cancer is the fastest-growing cancer in the world. MCP may one day help us slow the progress of this deadly disease. In a study reported in the *Journal of the National Cancer Institute* (March 18, pages 438-442, 1992), researchers induced skin cancer in mice. They found that when they also injected MCP, metastasis was decreased 90 percent. In those mice who did not receive MCP along with the cancer-causing substance, tumor colonies increased as much as 300 percent!

Immune function

A number of published papers show that MCP not only inhibits the growth and spread of cancer cells but also augments your body's natural immune response.

There is also evidence from tissue-culture studies, conducted at the Max Planck Institute in Tübingen, Germany, that modified citrus pectin can enhance the activity of the body's own killer cells.

Important note: Do not confuse MCP with natural citrus pectin (the kind that is commonly available in health-food stores). MCP has been tested extensively against natural citrus pectin, and the studies have shown that natural citrus pectin does NOT have the same immune boosting, cancer-killing effects.

To find out where you can obtain MCP, see A Guide to Sources and Availability, page 150. The recommended amount is 15 grams (or 3 rounded teaspoons) per day. Prices may vary but are usually lower when you buy in quantity. Expect to pay around $60 for 8 ounces.

Actions:
- Acts as an "antiadhesive agent" to prevent the cell interactions necessary for the transport and growth of tumor cells to secondary sites in the body
- Increases natural-killer-cell activity

Benefits:
- Naturally and specifically interferes with metastasis
- Augments the body's natural immune response

6

GLYCOALKALOIDS:
A NEW NON-SURGICAL SOLUTION FOR SKIN CANCER

Sooner or later, skin cancer affects nearly everyone. The removal of skin-cancer lesions is one of the most common outpatient surgeries performed today. But before you let your dermatologist schedule surgery to remove a cancerous or "suspicious" lesion, you should know about an inexpensive, all-natural product that can completely remove some skin cancers in as little as three to four weeks, without a trace of scar tissue.

You can also use this product to remove precancerous actinic keratoses (unsightly patches of scaly, sun-damaged skin that can turn cancerous at any time). Within a few weeks, any area of rough, uneven skin can be smoothed and renewed. (In fact, this cream is also being used to erase wrinkles, blemishes, and age spots—(more on that in a moment.)

The results are in: you can use this therapy with confidence

In recent months, you may have read of a natural botanical extract from Australia reported to be highly effective in treating skin cancers without surgery or harsh chemical treatments. We've received many letters from members asking for more information about the mysterious "devil's apple" plant and whether it is a safe and effective alternative for treating skin cancer.

There's no doubt that chemical compounds called glycoalkaloids, derived from the devil's apple

---

Depleted ozone levels leave you unprotected

This year, nearly 1 million cases of skin cancer will be diagnosed in the U.S. alone. Many scientists attribute rising skin cancer rates to the thinning of the ozone layer. Each 1% decrease in ozone translates into a 3% increase in the amount of UV-B radiation reaching the earth, which in turn translates into 10 to 15 thousand new cases of skin cancer. Experts predict that at this rate, worldwide skin cancer rates will be 26% higher in the year 2000 than they were in 1997.

plant, can effectively remove skin-cancer lesions. An Australian study of 72 patients posted a 100% cure rate. Unfortunately, there are drawbacks to the Australian product (although it is effective, it can be highly irritating to the skin and can take up to three months to work. Moreover, it is very difficult to obtain outside Australia.

Last year, however, a leading American research laboratory made several important advances in the formulation of glycoalkaloid cream. The researchers created a new product called SkinAnswer, which promised to be even more effective (and quicker) than the Australian prototype, and much less irritating to the skin.

And now, the first clinical trials on SkinAnswer are complete. The results have confirmed the preliminary reports beyond a doubt: It dissolves both basal cell and squamous-cell cancers in as little as three to four weeks, with absolutely no scarring. It also painlessly removes precancerous actinic keratosis lesions. Patients and doctors who have used both SkinAnswer and the earlier Australian version report that SkinAnswer seems to work more quickly and with less pain and irritation.

Selectively targets cancer cells; healthy cells are unaffected

Glycoalkaloids are produced in many fruits and vegetables as part of their defense against insects and other animals. Historically, the use of glycoalkaloid-rich plants (members of the Solanum family) in the treatment of cancer goes back to the second century.

As a treatment for skin cancer, glycoalkaloids are thought to work by exploiting structural differences between healthy and abnormal skin cells. As skin cells change from healthy to cancerous, the cell wall becomes more permeable, allowing glycoalkoloids to penetrate into abnormal cells. Once inside the cell wall, glycoalkaloids release enzymes that literally digest the cells from the inside out. Under a microscope, the cells actually appear to explode.

As the abnormal cells die, they are replaced by normal, healthy skin cells that do not absorb the glycoalkaloids and are spared their destructive effects.

In any cancer therapy, the ideal is a "targeted therapy"(one that attacks cancer cells and spares healthy ones. And it appears that SkinAnswer does precisely that. When it is applied to a cancerous lesion, you are likely to notice redness and inflammation(even a burning sensation (indicating that the cancer cells are being destroyed). An ulceration, or opening in the skin, may develop as the lesion begins to slough off.

These diseased cells will quickly be replaced by healthy cells, which are unaffected by the glycoalkaloid cream. In fact, you know that the treatment is complete when the cream no longer produces a reaction, indicating that normal healthy cells have replaced all of the skin-cancer cells.

For use on squamous cell or basal-cell skin cancers, SkinAnswer is applied to the area twice a day, as directed on the package. Before reapplying, rubbing the area with a washcloth to remove dead skin layers will speed the healing process. Treated areas should be left uncovered if at all possible. (Covering the treatment area with a bandage seems to increase the amount of irritation to the skin and may actually slow the speed of treatment.)

Get rid of that "suspicious" spot before it becomes cancerous

In addition to their dramatic effect on skin-cancer lesions, glycoalkaloids can also act a natural exfoliant that can smooth virtually any rough, uneven, or raised skin condition. As Dr. Margaret Olsen, author of the recent clinical trial, noted, "This study began as a search for treatment for basal and squamous cell cancers, but evolved into a more effective treatment for actinic [sun-damage-related] keratoses."

Several of the trial participants had, in addition to diagnosed skin cancers, extensive areas of sun damage, resulting in raised, scaly patches of actinic keratosis. According to Dr. Olsen, these patients came in for treatment for one or two symptomatic lesions, had thousands of keratosis lesions. They were, as Dr. Olsen noted, "generally oblivious to the extent of their sun damage."

Effectiveness of SkinAnswer in eliminating skin lesions

Type of lesion	Mean treatment	Complete period recovery
Basal cell	27 days	78%
Squamous cell	30 days	100%
Keratosis	31 days	72% (28% had partial recovery)

All results were confirmed by biopsy. In the cases in which only partial recovery was achieved in the trial period, it was anticipated that continued use would eventually result in 100% remission rates.

Source: Margaret Olsen, M.D., Chief of Dermatology at Saint John's Health Center, Santa Monica, California.

In addition to treating the active lesions as part of the trial, these patients also applied SkinAnswer to wide areas of sun-damaged skin. The result was easy and painless exfoliation of the keratoses, leaving smooth skin after a few weeks. These findings were confirmed by other researchers. With the ease and cost-effectiveness of SkinAnswer, there is no longer any reason to "watch and wait." Precancerous lesions can be removed immediately before the situation becomes more serious.

Other noncancerous, raised skin growths, such as moles, skin tags, and even "liver spots," can be effectively and painlessly removed by SkinAnswer's powerful exfoliating action. Although these irregularities usually pose no threat of cancer, you may wish to remove them for cosmetic reasons. Compared with elective cosmetic surgery, glykoalkaloids provide an extremely cost-effective alternative. Other treatment applications currently under investigation include acne and psoriasis.

Note: In the treatment of active lesions (basal-cell and squamous-cell cancers) with SkinAnswer, some temporary discomfort is to be expected. However, it appears to be far less uncomfortable than Efudex (commonly prescribed as a topical chemotherapy for skin cancers. One patient remarked, "If this were Efudex, I'd be screaming by now." In addition, SkinAnswer was effective on lesions that had been unsuccessfully treated with Efudex. SkinAnswer is essentially painless to use for keratoses and for other cosmetic applications.

A "face-lift in a jar?"

Dr. Allen Rosen, a prominent plastic surgeon in Bloomfield, New Jersey, began using SkinAnswer as part of a clinical trial for squamous-cell skin cancer. Like Dr. Olsen, he also found it to be highly effective in eroding noncancerous and precancerous lesions, such as keratoses. Its intense, yet gentle exfoliating action led Dr. Rosen to consider the role of glycoalkaloid creams as a treatment for fine lines and wrinkles. "Physician-administered glycolic peels are routinely used as an alternative to cosmetic surgery to rejuvenate the skin. SkinAnswer is an over-the-counter product that might be used in much the same way and with the same level of effectiveness [to reduce the effects of aging and sun exposure]. It has a gentleness that traditional peels do not have."

Dr. Rosen notes that the extent of exfoliation can be controlled through frequency of use and by covering the treatment area. He cautions against covering or bandaging the treatment area, as this can over-intensify the exfoliation effect, especially on delicate skin. Intense

> ### You can still enjoy the warm summer sun
> ### *(in fact, you should)*
>
> There are also some benefits to moderate sun exposure. For example, direct sunlight promotes the production of Vitamin D. Among its many beneficial functions, Vitamin D aids in the absorption of calcium, which is crucial to maintaining bone mass as we grow older. Unfortunately, our bodies make less vitamin D as we age. In fact, vitamin D deficiency is epidemic among seniors.
>
> Recent studies have shown that sufficient levels of antioxidant vitamins, like vitamin C, E, and betacarotene, act as natural sunscreens, protecting your skin from sunburns and other sun damage. (*Journal of Photochemistry and Photobiology*, vol. 41, nos. 1-2, pp. 1-10, 1997). So, take your antioxidants and enjoy a regular dose of sunlight. It will strengthen your bones and buoy your mood as well.

discomfort and/or burning may indicate a sensitivity or allergy to the product. In this case, use should be decreased or discontinued. (A slight tingling sensation when the cream is applied is normal.)

Dr. Rosen is now conducting a clinical trial on SkinAnswer as a cosmetic treatment for facial wrinkles and will have the results of that study by the end of the year. Although there is much research still to be done, he finds SkinAnswer to be "an incredibly exciting development in skin care."

It may be a year or more before the new clinical studies are published, but you or your doctor can request a set of the published glycoalkaloid research papers for $10 (including shipping) by calling 1(800)742-7534. SkinAnswer is available through some pharmacies and by mail order. (See page 148 for details.)

Actions:
- Penetrates into cancerous cells, where it releases enzymes that digest the cells from the inside out
- Acts as a powerful exfoliant

Benefits:
- Provides painless, cost-effective removal of precancerous growths and skin irregularities

7

PC SPES: "HOPE" FOR PROSTATE CANCER

In Chapter 16 of this book, we feature an innovative formulation of Chinese herbs called RA Spes that is extraordinarily effective in the treatment of rheumatoid arthritis. In the course of our research for that chapter, we came across another formulation by the same brilliant biochemist, Dr. Sophie Chen, called PC Spes. "PC" stands for prostate cancer, and spes is the Latin word for hope.

A blend of Chinese herbs, PC Spes dramatically extends and enhances the lives of prostate-cancer patients for whom traditional therapies have ceased to be effective, in some cases actually arresting and reversing the progression of the disease to other sites in the body. This little-known wonder is also being used to boost the effectiveness of other, more traditional, prostate-cancer therapies and is also recommended for those with early-stage prostate cancer who have been advised to "watch and wait."

A nontoxic alternative that is saving lives

PC Spes is an incredible breakthrough in the fight against prostate cancer, especially advanced cases. PC Spes not only is helpful as an adjunct therapy (in combination with other treatments) but also offers a new alternative when other treatments fail. Most importantly, it is adding years to the lives of men with hormonally refractive prostate cancer, who would otherwise be forced to submit to end-stage chemotherapy.

How does PC Spes work?

PC Spes is a combination of eight herbs seven from the realm of traditional Chinese medicine plus saw palmetto. As with all Chinese-medicine formulas, the combination of herbs is carefully designed to work synergistically—each herb being complemented and made more potent by the biologic actions of the others. Together, the herbs act on at least five levels: immune-stimulating, antitumor, antiviral, anti-inflammatory, and antibenign prostate hyperplasia.

> ### Let's define a few terms:
>
> **PSA: prostate specific antigen.** The presence of PSA in the blood can indicate the existence and extent of prostate cancer. The PSA test is used both as a routine screening test and to track the progression of the disease and the effectiveness of treatments employed. Prostate-cancer treatments aim to lower, or at least stabilize, PSA levels.
>
> **Gleason's score.** A microscopic analysis of prostate cells allows the doctor to assess the degree of malignancy present. A score of 1-4 indicates a low degree of cell mutation (or malignancy), 5-7 is considered moderate, and 8-10 denotes the highest degree of malignancy.
>
> **CHT: combination hormonal therapy.** A combination of two hormone "blockers" that starve the prostate tumor of the male sex hormones that spur its growth. Luteinizing hormone releasing hormone (LHRH agonist) is administered once a month by injection and blocks production of testosterone in the testes. A second antiandrogen is administered orally. The result is "chemical castration," and it is usually accompanied by side effects that include impotence, decrease in muscle mass, hot flashes, and pain. CHT has two uses: to shrink or "de-bulk" the diseased prostate in preparation for surgery or other treatments, and to slow the progression of advanced prostate cancer when other treatment options have been exhausted.
>
> **Hormone refractory:** Unfortunately, CHT is rarely a long-term solution. In a full 90 percent of cases, the disease eventually progresses to the extent that hormone therapy is no longer effective. At this point, the disease is classified as hormone refractory, and many physicians turn to chemotherapy as a last resort. While potent drugs can buy a little more time, the chemicals that are toxic to the cancer cells are ultimately toxic to the patient as well.

Recently published research indicates that the combination of standardized herbal extracts in PC Spes accelerates the rate of cell death (apoptosis). One way PC Spes does this is by interfering with a gene that normally protects cells from apoptosis. This suggests that PC Spes may also make cancer cells more responsive to other antitumor agents.

PC Spes also affects the receptors for male hormones, which in turn lowers PSA counts and slows the proliferation of prostate-cancer cells. Most significantly, it has the power to keep PSA counts down, even after the cancer has become hormonally refractive. At this stage, the patient typically has less than a year to live. For such patients, PC Spes can mean the difference between life and death, dramatically extending patients' lives and increasing their quality of life as well.

It is estimated that approximately 700 to 900 prostate-cancer patients have been treated with PC Spes. According to Dr. James Lewis Jr., author of *New Guidelines for Surviving Prostate Cancer*, PC Spes seems to have helped 70 percent of these patients, from those on watchful waiting to those undergoing chemotherapy.

Power herbs in PC Spes attack cancer on many levels

Isatis indigotica (da qing ye) contains beta-sitoterol, a phytosterol. Oral administration of beta-sitosterol is known to reduce tumor yield in animals with tumors.

Glycyrrhiza glabra and Glycyrrhiza uralensis (gan cao) contain saponins, which stimulate the immune system and possess anti-tumor activity in-vitro.

Glycyrrhiza also contains quercetin, which has demonstrated anti-tumor effects. In addition, glycyrrhiza lowers testosterone levels.

Panax pseudo-ginseng (san qi) enhances immunity by stimulating natural killer (NK) cell activity.

Ganoderma lucidum (ling zhi) contains polysaccharide compounds that markedly inhibit cancer cells and increase life span of test animals with lung cancers by up to 195%.

Scuterllaria baicalensis (huang qin) inhibits tumor-cell proliferation and encourages cell death (apoptosis). It also stimulates the immune system and has anti-bacterial actions.

Dendranthema morifolium Tzvel (Chu-hua) is a lesser-known Chinese herb with unspecified biologic effects. According to Chinese tradition, it is antiviral and detoxifying.

Rabdosia rebescens (don ling cau) has multiple anti-tumor effects and pain-relieving properties. Increased survival and reduced side effects from antineoplastic treatment has been noted in patients with cancer of the esophagus.

Saw palmetto decreases the bioavailability of testosterone and is frequently used in the treatment of benign prostatic hypertrophy.

Source: James Lewis, Jr. Ph.D., *New Guidelines for Surviving Prostate Cancer* Westbury, NY: Health Education Literary Publisher, 1998

Recently, PC Spes users gathered at a meeting of Man to Man, a prostate-cancer support group sponsored by the American Cancer Society, to share their individual experiences with fellow cancer patients. Here is just one brief excerpt from the transcript of this meeting:

> In 1991, I had a regular physical and there were two small bumps that showed up. My PSA was about 2.5, and the biopsy showed it was about a Gleason 3. Back then, there were not all the options that we have today. He [the urologist] was ready to get out his scalpel and go at it. So I went right along with it. I went through the operation fine...and then, about a year after the operation, [my PSA] started creeping up...bouncing around from 5 to 7. That's when the urologists say, 'Well, I don't really know what we're going to do for you.' It [PSA] finally reached 10.5 two months ago, and that's when I learned about PC Spes. The first month, it dropped down from 10.5 to 2.7. I just got my results back two days ago for the second month, and it's down to .07. I'm taking nine capsules a day...and so far it's been a miracle.

A lifesaving option in your hands

PC Spes is among the therapies that have not been approved by the FDA, but because it is a natural herbal preparation, it can be sold as a dietary supplement. Several forward-thinking oncologists are conducting clinical trials to further document the lifesaving actions of PC Spes. Studies are planned or under way at the Columbia Presbyterian Medical Center, at Sloan-Kettering Cancer Center in New York, and in sites around the country. Clinical testing is also being conducted at several hospitals in China.

Depending on the stage of the disease, the recommended protocol is between six and 12 capsules a day—at a cost of $300 to $600 a month. (Compare that to the price tag on CHT, which edges close to $10,000 a year.) PC Spes has been successfully used in combination with other therapies to boost effectiveness. For example, some practitioners find that by alternating PC Spes with CHT, they can delay the onset of the hormone-refractory phase of the disease.

For those with early-stage prostate cancer, who would normally be advised to "watch and wait," PC Spes can be used to lower PSA counts and then used at a lower dose (three capsules a day) to maintain those levels.

(Please note that cancer of any kind should always be treated in cooperation with a health professional.) Patients and doctors can request a comprehensive information packet on PC Spes from the Education Center for Prostate Cancer Patients P.O. Box 948, Westbury, NY 11590, tel. (516)997-1777, fax (516) 997-9555.

Because of its relatively short history, PC Spes must be considered an experimental therapy. It will be several years before long-term results are available, but, as Dr. Lewis notes, "PC Spes offers hope to thousands of prostate-cancer victims, extending their lives while the battle to find a cure rages on."

The Education Center for Prostate Cancer Patients publishes regular updates on PC Spes trials and protocols and also maintains a data base of complementary physicians who specialize in integrating natural and traditional therapies. Dr. Lewis' book titled *New Guidelines for Surviving Prostate Cancer*, in an updated 1998 edition, is also available from the same organization. PC Spes is available from the source listed on page 151.

Actions:
- Interferes with a gene that normally protects cancer cells from apoptosis
- Affects the receptors for male hormones

Benefits:
- May make cancer cells more responsive to other anti-tumor agents
- Lowers PSA counts and slows the proliferation of prostate-cancer cells
- Keeps PSA levels down even after the cancer has become hormonally refractive

8

Breast-cancer Detection: Making Breast Self-Exams Easier to Perform

Vast amounts of time, energy, and print have been devoted to establishing the age at which a woman should begin regular mammogram screening. Meanwhile, many experts agree that the real question isn't when or how often you should have one but whether you should have one at all. In other words, is mammography—at any age—worth the expense and risk?

False positives are just one of the risks

Routine mammograms done on women in their 40s are estimated to produce false positive results over a third of the time. That means that out of 10,000 women tested, 3,000 to 4,000 of them would have a mammogram falsely interpreted as "suspicious." And most of those women would have to undergo further testing to determine if their breasts were, in fact, normal. False positives result in anxiety, unnecessary biopsy procedures, scarring, and distortions of the breast, further straining the future accuracy of testing.

Even worse, spokespeople for the National Institutes of Health (NIH) admit that mammograms miss 25 percent of malignant tumors in women in their 40s (and 10 percent in older women). In fact, one Australian study found that more than half of the breast cancers in younger women are not detectable by mammograms.

These false negative results, which can lull women into a false sense of security, are equally as dangerous as false positives. In a study from Sweden in which women younger than 55 who had mammograms showed a 29 percent higher death rate from breast cancer, researchers said, "Although this could be a random phenomenon, negative results of a screening mammogram may have falsely reassured some patients and led to a deleterious delay in diagnosis."

And even if mammograms are accurately interpreted, consider this: The *New York Times* quotes Donald Berry, a Duke University statistician, as saying that "98.5 percent of women in their 40s will get no benefit" from mammograms. "The other 1.5 percent will have their lives extended by 200 days."

A deadly distraction...

Monica Miller, a government-relations specialist for alternative medicine, sees the whole debate about mammography as a deadly distraction from the abysmal state of breast-cancer care in the United States. Commenting on her personal choice to forgo mammogram screening, she says, "The idea of introducing radiation to radiation-sensitive tissue is absurd. If women start getting regular mammograms at 40, more cancers will be found because more cancers will be caused by the mammograms themselves."

A lot of sound and fury about one of the most questionable procedures in the fight against breast cancer.

The worst thing about the mammogram debate is the possibility that, in the resulting confusion, women will be more likely than ever to do

---

The evolution of an idea

In 1984, inventor Earl Wright was idly playing around with a half-deflated water balloon his grandson had left on the table. Rolling it back and forth over some grains of salt, it occurred to him that he could feel the salt right through the balloon—in fact, he could feel it better through the balloon!

Not yet sure of the possible applications of his discovery, Wright experimented with more than 80 combinations of different materials to find the one that enhanced his sense of touch the most. Then, he tried to figure out who might be helped by his new invention.

His first thought was to use it as an aid for reading Braille. People who are born blind learn this skill with relatively little difficulty. However, people who are newly blind often find it difficult to develop the fingertip sensitivity required for sightless reading. Earl went ahead with his plan to use his invention to help newly blind children and adults sensitize their fingers. And it worked. Still, he continued to search for other, broader uses.

When he realized its potential as an aid for breast self-examinations, the Sensor Pad was born. He reasoned that if the pad could increase the likelihood that a woman would correctly and regularly perform BSE, the odds of detecting and successfully treating early breast cancer would improve.

absolutely nothing to protect themselves. Attention has been diverted from the one procedure that allows women to take an active role in their own health care and that all experts agree is the key to the early detection of breast cancer: breast self-examinations (BSEs).

As one doctor puts it, "Women who do regular self-examinations can and do develop greater sensitivity toward their breasts and what is normal or abnormal than their doctors. In fact, between 50 and 60 percent of breast cancers are discovered by women themselves, either accidentally or through purposeful BSE."

There is an inexpensive and absolutely safe device that makes BSE much easier to perform and could increase its effectiveness. Unfortunately—and incomprehensibly—the FDA has refused to allow consumers direct access to this potentially lifesaving invention.

A maverick inventor's 11-year battle with the FDA

Earl Wright, an inventor from Decatur, Illinois, holds more than 150 U.S. and foreign patents. A former member of the U.S. Patent and Trademark Advisory Committee, he was named an Inventor of the Year finalist in 1989 for his development of the Sensor Pad in 1984.

The Sensor Pad is a simple, inexpensive device—a latex-like pad 9.5 inches in diameter filled with about 2 tablespoons of medical-grade liquid silicone that allows the two layers of the pad to slip smoothly over each other. When held over the breast during a BSE, it makes the fingertips more sensitive by reducing friction and magnifying sensation.

- The Sensor Pad makes it easier for women to learn proper BSE technique and, by reducing friction, makes it easier to detect changes in breast tissue.

- It gives women confidence in their own ability to perform these important monthly exams and acts as a visible reminder to do them regularly.

- For many older women who are uncomfortable touching their own bodies, the Sensor Pad provides an "indirect" way to examine themselves.

However, despite evidence from women who claim the Sensor Pad saved their lives, despite the professional testimony of doctors and other breast-cancer specialists who agree on the need for this product, and despite countless studies commissioned by the manufacturer showing it to be safe and effective, the FDA kept the Sensor Pad off the market in the United States for 11 years, citing a lack of scientific proof that the device works.

Is this consumer protection? Or a bureaucratic boondoggle?

In 1985, Earl and his son Grant were ready to market the Sensor Pad. They applied for authorization in Canada and got it within 30 days. They also got approval in Japan, Singapore, Korea, Thailand, and most West European countries. But when they asked the FDA for approval, they hit a roadblock.

The FDA kept asking for more and more information and more and more studies. "Ridiculous," says Grant Wright. "The Sensor Pad works on the same principle as soap and water—it reduces friction. Women are told to do breast exams using soap and water all the time. But you don't see the FDA asking for studies on that."

Still, the Wrights attempted to comply with request after request by the agency. They were especially frustrated because they didn't consider the Sensor Pad to be a medical device and therefore doubted that the FDA had any jurisdiction over it.

In 1988, after years of waiting, the Wrights consulted an attorney and were advised to start selling the pads directly to hospitals. The pads were enthusiastically accepted both by medical community and by patients. In little more than a year, the Wrights' company, Inventive

---

FDA classification keeps the Sensor Pad off the market

The FDA chose to classify the Sensor Pad as a "Class III medical device," a category that has included such invasive, high-tech inventions as pacemakers and heart-valve replacements—a category of products that, understandably, require extensive testing before FDA approval is given.

A Class III classification for the Sensor Pad? FDA spokesperson Sharon Snider defends this decision by insisting that the Sensor Pad poses an indirect threat. If it "fails to do what it's supposed to do," she says, "it could have very serious consequences for a woman: It could cost her her life."

However, no one is claiming that the Sensor Pad is anything more than a lubricating aid. Nancy G. Brinker, founder of the Susan G. Komen Breast Cancer Foundation, says, "There is no way you could convince me that doing a breast exam with a Sensor Pad could be any more harmful than not doing one at all—which is what happens with most women." She adds, "I think it's absolutely ridiculous that something that could be so potentially helpful to women is being kept off the market by government bureaucracy."

Products, sold more than 200,000 pads. Then, in 1991, the FDA got wind of this "unauthorized" activity and raided the company's headquarters, confiscated 30,000 pads, and, after a two-year legal battle, managed to bury the Sensor Pad even deeper in red tape.

Finally, a victory—of sorts

The Wrights didn't back down. They truly believed in their product, and so they continued to fight, spending millions of dollars in an effort to get FDA approval. Then just as they were about to give up, the FDA came through. Kind of.

The FDA finally approved the Sensor Pad in 1995, but only with a doctor's prescription. Their reasoning for restricting sales was to ensure that a certified physician would show a woman the proper way to use the pad, and ensure that it would not replace regular mammograms.

Unfortunately, the FDA's approval put such limitations on acquiring the Sensor Pad that a woman could not even get the prescription filled at a pharmacy. It had to be done directly through her doctor's office. In addition, the FDA even went as far to disallow the Wrights to mass-market the pad to hospitals and health maintenance organizations. This was an expensive setback for the Wrights, and there was concern that doctors would be less likely to order the pad due to their liability for items that require a prescription.

The FDA's ruling started an onslaught of letters and calls outraged that they would require a prescription for a non-prescription product. After two more years of inquiries and protests, the FDA finally approved over the counter sales of the Sensor Pad in 1997. But due to the small size of the Wright's company, and all costs accrued since the breast pad's development 14 years prior to the ruling, an attempt at mass-marketing was too expensive for the Wrights to front on their own.

Then in 1998, Wright's Inventive Products Corporation reached a marketing agreement with B-D, Inc. (formerly Becton Dickinson) concerning the promotion and production of the breast pad. After that agreement was made, and with a subtle name change, the Sensability Pad became readily available to the general public. Remarkably since B-D, Inc. has added the Sensability Pad onto its list of products, the FDA hasn't protested its widespread accessibility.

Currently, the Sensability Pad can be purchased without a prescription through the Internet and in national drug store chains like Wal-Mart, Walgreens, K-Mart, and Eckerd's, as well as through your doctor's office. The breast pad comes with a videotape and instruction manual that emphasizes the need for professional breast exams and mammograms, as well as monthly self-exams.

Actions:
- Works on the same principle as soap and water, making fingertips more sensitive by reducing friction and magnifying sensation.

Benefits:
- Makes it easier for women to learn the proper BSE technique
- Makes it easier to detect changes in breast tissue

9

PHYTOCHEMICALS: NATURE'S "SUPER FOODS"

There's no doubt that certain natural substances found in many plants-called phytochemicals—have the power to keep you well. Medical literature is saturated with epidemiological studies showing a direct correlation between low levels of plant foods in the diet and high rates of disease and untimely death.

In one of the largest and longest-running studies, researchers at the Institute of Preventive Oncology in Tokyo proved, once and for all, that your diet—specifically, the amount of fruits and vegetables you regularly eat—is the primary factor in predicting health and longevity.

Phytochemicals give a plant its color, flavor, and smell, but more importantly, they are part of a plant's natural defense system. Researchers have found that these same protective qualities can also boost your body's disease-fighting, detoxifying, and antiaging abilities. And, because of our increasing exposure to toxins in our food, water supply and environment, these natural substances are increasingly crucial to our physical well-being.

While the benefits are clear, research shows that Americans on the average eat only 25% to 35% of the five to six recommended daily servings of fruits and vegetables. Realistically, consuming five to six servings is hard to do. That's at least two servings of vegetables and fruit at every meal, and you have to vary the plants you eat to get all the important nutrients you need.

Furthermore, what we do eat is usually cooked, canned, or frozen (neutralizing up to 90% of the vital nutrients). Fortunately, extensive research has pinned down the best sources of these phytochemicals and is now heralding them as being among our best nutritional defenses against our toxic, disease-promoting environment and lifestyles.

The broccoli breakthrough

In 1992, Dr. Paul Talalay's laboratory at Johns Hopkins University isolated a chemical in broccoli called sulforaphane. Also found in kale, cabbage, and cauliflower, sulforaphane activates Phase II enzymes, which are responsible for breaking down and eliminating highly reactive compounds that are known to damage DNA and ultimately set the stage for the cancer process.

In 1997, after testing broccoli at different stages of growth, Dr. Talalay's team of researchers determined that 3-day-old broccoli sprouts contain amazingly high levels of sulforaphane-from 30-50 times the concentration found in mature broccoli plants. In controlled studies, the broccoli-sprout extract significantly reduced the size and amount of breast tumors in lab animals exposed to a known carcinogen.

The power of an ancient Asian panacea

Green tea is not only a popular beverage in Asia but also a regularly prescribed medicine. It is made by lightly steaming the fresh-cut C. Sinesus leaf, yielding a nontoxic unfermented tea "alive" with a group of active photochemicals called polyphenols. Polyphenols have been rigorously studied and proven to do all of the following:

- increase the body's ability to use and eliminate unhealthy (LDL) cholesterol
- block the tumor-promoting action of nitrosamines and other dietary carcinogens that are generated during the curing or cooking of fish, meats, and vegetables
- supercharge the enzyme activity of your organs—especially the liver, lungs, and small intestine—to detoxify and cleanse away free radicals and other toxins
- protect the lungs from potent toxins found in tobacco protect you with antioxidant power that's 20 times more powerful than vitamin E

And it does much more: Green-tea extract has also been shown to protect lab animals from cancer-cell growth in the colon, mammary tissue, and stomach; reduce the risk to blood clots by inhibiting the clotting factor called thomboxane A2 (via the same method by which aspirin works); protect the skin from UV radiation; act as a natural ACE inhibitor to lower blood pressure; reduce blood-sugar levels; and even kill oral bacteria that can cause cavities and bad breath.

Clearly, certain phytochemicals are more directly beneficial to human health, and science has begun to establish a team of phytochemical "all-stars." For maximum protection against cancer, heart disease, and other degenerative diseases, be sure to eat plenty of grapes, ginger, tomatoes, and turmeric, in addition to broccoli and green tea.

Grape-skin extract: the "one-in-a thousand" cell protector. Resveratrol, the phytochemical in grape skin (and red wine) enables the French, well known for their high-fat diet, to have such low heart-disease rates. Resveratrol is now famous for its ability to protect the heart-but it does more than that: It also has been shown in studies to block tumor growth and the production of abnormal cells.

Ginger: even better for your blood than garlic. Best known for its ability to treat motion sickness, nausea, and vomiting, ginger is a very powerful antioxidant, a little-known but highly effective pain reliever, an anti-inflammatory, a cholesterol lowering agent, and even a cardiotonic. When taken regularly, it helps prevent ulcers, ensures healthy digestive functioning, and even prevents infection.

Lycopcene: The "tomato antioxidant" that protects your entire body. Lycopene is the pigment that gives tomatoes, apricots, watermelon, and red grapefruit their deep, rich color...and is the phytochemical responsible for the exciting results of the now famous Harvard study (of over 48,000 men!) showing that tomatoes protect one's prostate health. It's also a superior antioxidant that can protect your cells from damage and mutation.

Tumeric: An ancient spice, dye, and preservative, and medicine, turmeric was a staple of Greek herbal medicine, and it is still used today in traditional Chinese and Indian medicine to treat a mind-boggling array of conditions, including liver disorders, chest pain, menstrual disorders, inflammation, eczema, and hemorrhage! Curcumin, the phytochemical in turmeric, increases bile-acid output, which provides tremendous aid in the processing of fats and fat-soluble nutrients, and increases the elimination of cholesterol from your system.

Variety is the spice of life

Modify your diet to include as many of these phytochemical-rich sources as possible. Don't forget to also increase the amount of fruits and vegetables you currently consume. If you're bored with the same old assortment, visit a local market and discover that there are probably dozens of fruits and vegetables that you've never even tried. Try to incorporate these novel and exotic varieties into your diet by experimenting with new recipes. Don't neglect your old stand-bys, but remember this: the more diverse your selection, the more types of phytochemicals you will be consuming.

If you find it difficult to eat the recommended variety or quantity of phytochemical-rich fruits and vegetables, don't worry. Phytochemical supplements are available from several manufacturers. The best products include a synergistic combination of several complementary phytonutrients like those listed above. Check labels to ensure standardized potencies. A high-quality phytonutrient product is available from the source listed on page 151.

Actions:
- Acts as a powerful antioxidants
- Acts as a detoxifying agent
- Acts as an anti-inflammatory
- Acts as an anticarcinogenic
- Promotes antiaging

Benefits:
- Support the immune system to help detect and kill tumors, lower LDL cholesterol, lower blood pressure, neutralize free radicals, and detoxify the system.

SECTION III
A Strong Heart for the Next Century

One in every 2.4 Americans dies from heart disease. Even though "only" one in every four Americans today has any of the symptoms—chest pain, high blood pressure, or exertion pain...almost every man and woman in America has some degree of heart disease. The cholesterol-lowering drugs you're currently taking may not be doing enough to protect the health of your heart and cardiovascular system—in fact, cholesterol is not the enemy the medical establishment once thought it was! Take steps now to boost your circulation, lower your homocysteine levels, and harness the power of an amazing "entrainment" technique for your heart. See also the chapter on Larreastat (page 91) for another way to naturally fortify your heart.

10

Cardiocysteine: Reduce Your Risk of Heart Disease

Whether you know it or not, you may already have heart disease. And you won't find the total protection you need in a garlic or fish-oil capsule...any more than you'll find it in a beta-blocker or calcium channel blocker. Neither will you find protection in the ever-popular low-fat diets.

All around the world, crossing genetic and environmental borders, cultures with exceptionally low rates of heart disease have enjoyed and continue to enjoy diets loaded with high-fat, high-cholesterol foods—from the French, with their high-fat cheeses and butter sauces, to the people from northern India, for whom butter makes up a very high percentage of their daily calories!

And that's to say nothing of the Myskoke, a group of American Indians, and many other nonindustrialized populations, such as the Eskimos, who consume huge amounts of dietary cholesterol—and have high blood cholesterol—but have very low rates of death from heart disease.

Cholesterol is not the villain

The simple truth is that cholesterol is not the deadly threat you may think it is! Aside from the fact that it is necessary for everything from the production of sex hormones to bile synthesis...it simply does not clog up your arteries unless it has something to attach to: a tear, a rough surface, a ridge, or a sharp turn.

On that ridge or bump, cholesterol, blood products, and calcium begin to accumulate. These are the blood traps that lead to such problems as impotence, poor memory, heart attacks, strokes, and even death.

Harvard's "underground" theory of heart disease

Over 30 years ago, Dr. Kilmer McCully initiated the research that eventually led to the biggest breakthrough in the treatment and prevention of heart disease of our time. McCully, a professor at Harvard

Medical College, was researching the causes of arteriosclerosis—then, as now, the No.1 killer of both men and women in America. Dr. McCully suspected that something critical was missing from the mainstream theory on heart disease and, in 1969, proposed the first homocysteine theory of that ailment.

Thirty years and hundreds of studies later, we now know that there is a definite link between homocysteine levels in the blood and heart disease.

Homocysteine can kill—if you don't know how to control it

Your body forms homocysteine when you eat food containing an amino acid called methionine, which is present in all animal and vegetable protein. As part of the digestive process, methionine is broken down into homocysteine. As long as certain helper nutrients are present, homocysteine converts back to methionine, or to another amino acid called cystathionine. (Both are harmless.)

Early research showed that vitamin B_6 is one of the key helper nutrients necessary for normalizing homocysteine levels. When B_6 is low in the blood, homocysteine is high. Unfortunately, the typical American diet is low in vitamin B_6 and high in methionine. And because of food processing, it's virtually impossible to get adequate B_6 in the North American diet.

As McCully discovered early on in his research, homocysteine is even deadlier than had been imagined. It knocks out a mechanism in your artery cells, called "contact inhibition," that keeps the smooth muscle cells just below the inner wall of the artery from growing too rapidly.

At this stage, the smooth muscle cells begin multiplying too fast—just as some forms of cancer do! This creates a bulge that pushes other cells apart and protrudes into the artery, making atherosclerosis possible. The inner wall becomes uneven and rough at this spot, and the buildup of plaque begins.

McCully went even further to suggest that fat in the diet is only a "secondary complication" and that homocysteine overload is the "initial pathogenic factor." Simply put...you should be just as concerned—if not more so—over your homocysteine level as you are over your cholesterol level!

Since McCully first proposed his theory on heart disease, the evidence has mounted little by little, showing that...McCully was right all along!

A team of Seattle researchers showed that injections of homocysteine rapidly caused early signs of arteriosclerosis in baboons. The researchers reported that the cells just beneath the artery wall were mutating and reproducing at a wild rate and that this wild growth was destroying the arterial wall! After just one week of high levels of homocysteine in the baboons' blood, they lost 23 percent of their artery walls. The researchers found that the higher the level of homocysteine and the more severely injured the inner artery wall, the more severe the signs of arteriosclerosis. Again: Cholesterol levels were not correlated to the destruction of the arteries; cholesterol levels were secondary!

In another study, researchers at the University of Wisconsin's department of nutritional science studied the connection between methionine and B_6 in the diet. For the first 14 days, they gave six male subjects a high-protein diet, supplemented with 2 milligrams of B_6 a day. During that time, they found no homocysteine in the urine of the subjects. The researchers then took away the B_6 supplements but kept the high-protein diet the same. By the 21st day, all six men had high levels of homocysteine in their urine.

At the end of the 21-day period, the B_6 supplements (2 milligrams per day) were added back into the diet, and the homocysteine levels

Homocysteine and Alzheimer's Disease

In recent months, several unpublicized studies have revealed startling new links among homocysteine levels, B vitamins, and age-related cognitive decline. The first clue came in 1996, when a study of elderly Americans found that those with high homocysteine levels performed more poorly on certain cognitive tests. Researchers also noted that those with lower levels of vitamin B_{12} and folic acid showed reduced mental performance (*American Journal of Clinical Nutrition*, vol. 63, PP. 306-14, 1996).

Then in 1997, a six-year study revealed that subjects who supplemented with B_6 and B_{12} performed better on cognitive tests, including recall ability (*Am. Journal of Clinical Nutrition*, vol. 65, pp. 20-29, 1997). And most recently a Belgian study found that patients with Alzheimer's disease have higher levels of homocysteine in their blood (*Gerontology and Biological Science*, vol. 52, no. 2, pp. M76-9, 1997).

Homocysteine is a killer in more ways than ever suspected. Taking an antihomocysteine not only is great insurance against heart disease but also can help you preserve peak mental functioning as you age.

dropped dramatically in all participants.

It didn't end with B_6. Other researchers uncovered similar links between homocysteine and folic acid and between homocysteine and B_{12}, and they found that you need all three nutrients to keep homocysteine levels down.

A study at the Titus County Memorial Hospital, Mount Pleasant, Texas, showed that high homocysteine levels are a risk factor for atherosclerosis and that atherosclerosis is strongly associated with deficiencies of vitamin B_6, folate, and cobalamin (B_{12}). In that study, the patients who were given vitamin B_6 alone were able to reduce their risk of chest pain and heart attack by 73 percent vs. those who did not add B_6. Those who took B_6 lived an average of eight years longer than those who didn't.

You can't ensure healthy, effective levels of B_6, B_{12} and folic acid through diet alone. B_6, for example, is destroyed by heating, dehydration, and all other types of food processing.

Frighteningly, 80 percent of food consumed by Americans is processed. The average loss of B_6 from freezing fruits and fruit juices is about 15 percent, and from canning, it's 38 percent. Processed and refined grains lose 51 to 94 percent. Processed meats—which are high in methionine—lose 50 to 75 percent. Food processing causes comparable losses of folic acid and B_{12}.

Americans are so deficient in these nutrients that even the Food and Drug Administration (FDA) and the Centers for Disease Control (CDC) have stepped in to launch campaigns to get you to increase your intake through supplementation.

Unfortunately, we've discovered that most multivitamin formulas fall short. They simply don't have enough B_6, B_{12}, or folic acid to be effective in reducing your homocysteine levels.

There is one high-quality supplement, called Cardiocysteine Formula, that is based on the latest homocysteine research. Each tablet provides 800 mcg of folic acid, 500 mcg of B_{12} and 25 mcg of B_6. In addition, the formula includes 5 mg of pyridoxal-5-phosphate and 250 mg of trimethylglycine to ensure proper absorption and to boost the metabolism of homocysteine. See the "Guide to Sources and Availability" on page 147 for availability.

A final word of caution

We are not saying that homocysteine overload is the only cause of heart disease. There may be other ways in which atherosclerosis is initiated. But all the evidence is there for your scrutiny. You can drastically decrease the likelihood of atherosclerosis by adding to your daily regimen nutrients designed to reverse homocysteine levels in your blood.

Actions:
- Lowers serum homocysteine
- Ensures proper absorption to boost metabolism of homosysteine

Benefits:
- Reduces the risk of heart disease and atherosclerosis
- Increase peak mental function as you age

11

Freeze-Frame®: 60 Seconds to a Longer Life

As you know, the very first symptom of heart disease can be death. In the face of this grim reality, we're thrilled to be able to share with you an exciting new development in cardiology research. The Institute of HeartMath®, a nonprofit educational and research corporation, has developed an assessment tool that helps doctors identify candidates for sudden cardiac death. Its research has also led to a technique that you can use. Not only can it help reverse existing hypertension, but it may also lower the chance of sudden cardiac death.

HeartMath® has assembled an international team of superstars in the fields of cardiology, neurology, immunology, quantum physics, and psychology. These scientists have pioneered new biomedical research showing a direct relationship between mental/emotional balance and the healthy functioning of your heart, hormonal system, and immune system. They've unraveled the mystery of "entrainment," a natural phenomenon that occurs when two or more rhythmic systems, such as heartbeats and brain waves, synchronize.

Using the power of entrainment, HeartMath® has developed a tool so powerful that the U.S. military is having its personnel trained in it. Heads of corporations are footing the bill for their employees, and alternative-health practitioners are flocking to HeartMath's training center in Boulder Creek, California.

This five-step process, called Freeze-Frame®, creates entrainment within your nervous system, producing proven results unlike those of any other self-relaxation method. At first, HeartMath® taught the technique only in special seminars conducted at the Institute in Boulder Creek. But it became clear that Freeze-Frame® was extraordinarily effective, not only in lowering blood pressure but also in managing depression and anxiety, improving immune response, and providing other health benefits. So HeartMath® produced a special videotape program of the method, which you can use in your own home.

When you first learn how to do Freeze-Frame®, you might wonder how something so simple could possibly work, but don't be fooled. This is powerful stuff. One Fortune 100 company sent its employees—executives, administrative personnel, engineers, and factory workers alike—to learn this simple, straightforward technique. At the start of the study, 26 percent of the executive group had high blood pressure. Six months later, they all had normal readings. Even more astonishing, many reported the disappearance of long-standing symptoms like insomnia, headaches, indigestion, heartburn, and rapid heartbeat.

With Freeze-Frame®, you "remove yourself" from your disruptive feelings, relax, focus, and entrain your heart rhythms, respiration, and blood pressure, all in five simple steps. Think of great athletes or dancers who are able to create a special, relaxed state of mental and physical focus in order to achieve a much higher level of performance. Now you can employ that exact principle with any mental or emotional activity. And the benefit to your heart is phenomenal.

Outsmart your body's primitive "fight or flight" responses

Using this new HeartMath® technology, you can gain control of your autonomic nervous system—right down to the hormones you produce and the beat of your heart. With Freeze-Frame®, you learn to induce entrainment, in which your entire system—heart, glands, organs, and nervous system—works at maximum efficiency. It's no coincidence that moments of entrainment are associated with a deep sense of peace, fulfillment, and joy.

The results of HeartMath's research, published in the *American Journal of Cardiology*, the *Journal of Alternative Therapies*, and *Stress Medicine*, demonstrate conclusively that Freeze-Frame can significantly lower stress and may reduce your risk of sudden cardiac death. Case studies are showing blood pressure restored to normal levels. And there are many more reported benefits, including increased energy and mental clarity, improved immune response, and relief from the symptoms of chronic fatigue and certain autoimmune diseases.

Some day, perhaps all forms of hypertension—and many other diseases—will be healed with powerful heart-mind-body techniques like Freeze-Frame®, instead of dangerous drugs and surgery. This is a medicine of the future—available today.

In addition to offering the Freeze-Frame® program, Planetary

Publications offers HeartMath® books, audiocassettes, videotapes, and other educational materials, as well as original musical recordings scientifically demonstrated to improve hormonal, emotional, and immune-system balance. For more information, see page 148 for the "Guide to Sources and Availability."

Actions:
- balances your automatic nervous system to work at maximum efficiency
- puts your whole body into a more efficient balance

Benefits:
- help to reverse existing hypertension
- lower chance of cardiac death
- facilitates healing of cardiovascular diseases.

12

ORGANIC GERMANIUM: "ELECTRIFY" YOUR HEALTH

Supercharged mineral discovered! In 1886, a German chemist discovered an unidentified chemical—a mineral occurring in small quantities in foods, coal deposits, and the earth's crust. He called the substance "germanium." In 1950, Dr. Kazuhiko Asai, a brilliant Japanese chemist, discovered traces of germanium in fossilized plants. The next news about germanium came from Russia, where reports suggested that it had anticancer properties.

A few years later, Dr. Asai discovered that many healing plants—such as garlic, aloe, comfrey, chlorella, ginseng, shiitake mushrooms, and watercress—have significant concentrations of germanium. The holy water of Lourdes, known for its therapeutic value, also contains germanium.

In 1967, Dr. Asai managed to synthesize a new compound of germanium and found that the manufactured substance also had amazing curative abilities!

This product has come to be known as "organic germanium." (You may wonder how something man-made can be called "organic." The reason is that anything containing carbon in its molecular architecture is organic. Thus, synthetically derived germanium is, according to definition, organic.)

How does germanium "electrify" your health?

If you are old enough to have assembled a crystal radio in your youth, you may remember the germanium diode crystal, which was responsible for bringing in the radio signal that you heard in your earphone. The germanium atom is so structured that it accepts and transmits electrons, giving it a semiconductor capability. This means it becomes an electrostimulator, inducing the flow of electricity. In its pure metallic form, germanium is used extensively in the electronics industry for transistors, fiber optics, and other diverse applications.

Biologically, it appears to be able to stimulate electrical impulses on a cellular level. Science has established—as undisputed fact—that our bodies, our nerves, and our muscles are all electrically linked. So any substance that can enhance our electrical "connections" is bound to have a profound and life-giving effect.

Germanium has several unique and extremely valuable properties. It acts as:

- **an oxygen enhancer:** It has been shown to increase the flow of oxygen to all cells, especially in those areas that suffer from poor circulation.
- **a detoxifier:** Because of its chemical structure, germanium tends to bind or chelate (grab) and then remove toxic compounds and harmful substances from your system.
- **an adaptogen:** It "normalizes" your body's functions and adjusts to your specific needs. In the case of cancer, for example, it doesn't kill the cancer cells directly but stimulates your immune defenses to produce the substance that will, in turn, help to destroy the antagonist.
- **an immune catalyst:** Germanium helps to convert inactive macrophages—important immune cells—to active cells. It also enhances interferon production and increases natural killer cells.
- **a brain booster:** It has been reported to increase mental capacity, possibly because it helps your body send oxygen to the delicate tissues of the brain.

But even after 20 years of clinical and lab research, germanium is still virtually unknown in the United States. It remains a "mysterious" healing substance. Unfortunately, it takes many years from the time a discovery is recognized to the time when its importance is truly understood and accepted. In fact, medical historians inform us that the average delay from journal reporting to actual clinical use can be 50 or more years!

Ironically, the better a substance works...the more difficult it is to convince the mainstream medical community of its value. If a manufacturer wants the FDA to evaluate germanium and approve it for specific usage, it will have to show precisely how it works. But germanium appears to have endless curative abilities. Even if we had the technology and know-how to explain its various actions, it could still take decades to prove each application to the FDA.

Nevertheless, germanium works. And you can use it today! For prevention, one 150-milligram capsule daily is generally recommended.

In the presence of serious illness, physicians often recommend from 500 to 2,000 milligrams (2 grams) daily. Some manufacturers supply germanium by the kilo, at a substantial savings. For purchasing information, see the "Guide to Sources and Availability" on page 151.

Actions:
- Binds to toxins and metals so that they are easily removed
- Increases oxygen flow and uptake throughout your body
- Enhances interferon production
- Normalizes and balances bodily functions like blood pressure and immune-system activity

Benefits:
- Promotes quick healing through better circulation
- Promotes quick pain relief
- Helps prevent circulation problems
- Boosts energy and mood

SECTION IV
New Solutions for Autoimmune Diseases

Nature supplies us with many potent and nontoxic solutions to the illnesses and conditions that we struggle with every day. If you are among the millions who live with arthritis, herpes, or osteoporosis...and have felt let down by the "solutions" that traditional medicine has to offer—you'll find both help and hope in the pages that follow. Go beyond traditional painkillers that just mask the pain and discover natural products that can halt bone loss, grow new cartilage, control the debilitating pain of arthritis, and put an end to herpes breakouts.

See the chapters on infopeptides (page 13) and natural progesterone cream (page 121) for other important breakthroughs that can ease the pain and discomfort of arthritis and protect against osteoporosis.

13

Thymic Formula: Reverse Hepatitis, Rheumatoid Arthritis, and More

When rumors spread that a small-town doctor was curing patients of "incurable" hepatitis infections, Dr. Michael Rosen, then a medical correspondent for an Atlanta, Georgia, television station, went to Savannah to investigate. Although he originally planned an exposé on "quack" medicine, Dr. Rosen ended up filming an enthusiastic multipart report on Dr. Carson Burgstiner and his breakthrough method for treating so-called "incurable" diseases. Outside the local viewing area, however, Dr. Burgstiner's discovery remains largely unknown.

What caused Dr. Rosen's unexpected conversion? An impressive body of evidence in the form of Burgstiner's patients and their stories. In his own clinical experience, Dr. Burgstiner had witnessed the following:

> 84 cases of hepatitis B arrested
> 34 cases of hepatitis C arrested
> 28 cases of rheumatoid arthritis arrested
> 12 cases of systemic lupus in remission
> 10 cases of multiple sclerosis arrested
> 12 cases of psoriasis arrested

Whatever other therapies were employed, Dr. Burgstiner's treatment protocol featured the same "magic bullet" in every case. He had, over years of experimentation and analysis, identified a specific combination of nutrients, including extract of thymic glandular tissues, that appeared to stimulate his patients' malfunctioning immune systems and reverse even supposedly incurable conditions. The news spread from one cured patient to the next, and a steady stream of hopeful patients began trickling into Savannah to see Dr. Burgstiner.

The most impressive case history in Burgstiner's files may be his own

Burgstiner was a board-certified obstetrician-gynecologist, a past president of the Medical Association of Georgia, and a fellow of several prestigious medical associations. In 1983, He contracted hepatitis B when he punctured his finger while operating on an infected patient. The acute infection progressed to chronic illness, and Dr. Burgstiner, then a carrier of the blood-borne virus, was forced to limit his practice to nonsurgical procedures.

After seven years, Burgstiner was still sick and was frustrated at his body's inability to heal itself. His search for answers led him to focus on the role of the thymus gland in controlling the immune system. Unique among all the glands of the human body, the thymus reaches its maximum size in childhood, when it weighs up to 2 ounces. In early adulthood, the thymus begins to shrink; it eventually stops functioning altogether and withers to a few grams of shriveled tissue.

Recalling the medical principle of using glandular extracts to supplement underfunctioning glands like the thyroid and pancreas, Dr. Burgstiner reasoned that supplementing with thymus extract might restore his malfunctioning immune system. As he explained: "If your thyroid dries up, we give you thyroid. If your pancreas dries up, we give you insulin. If your ovaries dry up, we give you female hormones. However, when the thymus gland dries up, no one treats that as a medical condition, even though every doctor and nurse is taught that the thymus gland controls the immune system."

As HSI panelist Dr. Michael Rosenbaum explains in his book, *Super Supplements* (with Dominick Bosco, Signet, pp. 65, 83, 1989);

"Glandular extracts were among the original cornerstones of medicine, and were first used many thousands of years ago. Most ancient cultures, from the Egyptians, to the Hindus, to the Greeks, used glandular therapy. Among the glandular supplements, thymus substance is the most important. You want all the possible rejuvenation of the thymus gland that you can get, because the thymus gland is the major controlling gland of the immune system."

Dr. Burgstiner purchased thymic extract and a vitamin-mineral complex from a local health-food store and began taking them. Six weeks later, after seven years of chronic infection, his blood test for the hepatitis virus was negative. Amazed, he reported his results to the authorities. The Centers for Disease Control in Atlanta, the Massachusetts General Hospital in Boston, and the Scripps Institute in California all confirmed his test results, proclaiming him to have undergone a "spontaneous remission." Dr. Burgstiner's surgical privileges were restored.

The balance of Dr. Burgstiner's career was dedicated to the research, refinement, and documentation of the near-miraculous results he and scores of patients experienced using this thymic protocol. An independent laboratory tested the supplements and confirmed that they produced marked increases (up to 700 percent) in immune-system activity, as measured by the levels of thymic hormones in the blood.

Specific nutrients provide key activating agents

Further research established that the thymic extract alone, without the vitamin and mineral formula, did not have the same effect. Dr. Burgstiner theorized that the nutrients provided key activating agents for the natural synthesis of immune factors. Patients were dispatched to the health-food store with a shopping list for the various nutrients and instructions for the complicated regimen. Over the following years, Dr. Burgstiner fine-tuned his protocol, searching for ways to maximize its effectiveness.

Ultimately, he joined forces with a manufacturer to produce what he felt would be the most effective combination of nutrients, minimizing the expense and inconvenience for his patients. The final formulation included thymic factors and other glandular extracts, antioxidants, amino acids, enzymes, herbs, and minerals. (The only complaint ever registered by his patients was that the pills are somewhat large.)

Dr. Burgstiner's practice, once primarily obstetrics and gynecology, was transformed into a practice treating patients with a wide variety of immune-related conditions. Burgstiner felt that his thymic formula produced an immune-regulating effect—that is, in hyperimmune conditions, such as rheumatoid arthritis and multiple sclerosis, it would turn the overactive immune response down. In hypoimmune conditions like cancer, it would turn the immune response up.

Some of Dr. Burgstiner's colleagues are now recommending his thymic formula to their own patients. Susan Kolb, M.D., reports as follows: "I put all my patients on [Burgstiner's] Thymic Formula before and after surgery. They feel much better, recover quicker, and have fewer symptoms. They have increased energy levels, fewer muscular aches, and lower infection rates."

HSI panelist Ann Louise Gittleman, M.S., C.N.S., is also quite impressed with the formula: "I have found Burgstiner's Thymic Formula to be very helpful, particularly for my readers who needed special nutritional support for hepatitis C and other immune-related disorders. In my own research, I have found the glandular extracts to represent the true fountain of youth."

There are, however, many in the conventional medical community who question Burgstiner's theory. Some argue that it is normal for the thymus to stop functioning, simply because it is no longer needed. As Dr. Burgstiner's case files swelled with miraculous cures and remissions, the next step was to pursue large-scale, double-blind trials that would document his results to the satisfaction of the skeptics.

Unfortunately, Dr. Burgstiner died before he was able to see his theory proven and fully recognized. But the formula he created survives him, and the momentum of his incredible discovery continues. The National Institute of Health and the Centers for Disease Control have both expressed interest in investigating Dr. Burgstiner's Thymic Formula. Trials are planned or under way at the University of Alabama-Birmingham and Nova Southeastern University.

Meanwhile, as Dr. Burgstiner told Dr. Rosen, to wait for the research to be complete would mean that many would miss the opportunity to get well. Dr. Rosen, originally expecting to debunk Dr. Burgstiner's claims, has become a champion of the formula. As he commented in his report, "Is thymic extract a hidden hope for good health, or are Dr. Burgstiner's many patient testimonials the result of a placebo effect? I interviewed patients from diverse backgrounds and geographic locales, with a variety of different illnesses, all of whom have reached the same conclusion: If this is a placebo effect, it is an amazing one!"

Dr. Burgstiner's Thymic Formula continues to be manufactured and distributed from his home state of Georgia. All of the individual components in the formula have been completely evaluated for safety and meet FDA standards. Although most of the constituents—including the thymic extract—can be found in health-food stores, as single nutrients and in various combinations, Burgstiner's extensive work with his formula demonstrated that its potent effect relies on this particular combination and dosage.

The formula provides excellent and multifaceted nutritional support when taken as a daily vitamin-mineral-herbal supplement. For this purpose, the recommended dosage is six tablets per day. The therapeutic, immune-enhancing protocol used in most of the cases cited above calls for 12 tablets a day. Before adding the Thymic Formula to your current supplement regimen or medications, however, please consult your personal physician for advice.

Dr. Burgstiner's patients report that, in general, they experienced a significant improvement within 30 days. Dr. Rosen will soon be publishing a book about Dr. Burgstiner and his remarkable story.

Reports from grateful patients

"I had hepatitis C, and Thymic Formula cleared up my liver-function tests. I think I can live forever with this liver. My disease has been cured."

—Tony P.

"I have multiple sclerosis. My symptoms cleared up completely after beginning Thymic Formula."

—Pat M.

"I had hepatitis B and was given no hope. Two months after beginning Thymic Formula, my blood work showed no hepatitis B virus in my system. Without a shadow of a doubt, the Thymic Formula saved my life."

—Cynthia F.

"I had lupus and could not get out of bed. My kidneys became involved, and I was spilling blood and protein in my urine. Five days after beginning Thymic Formula, my energy level was normal and my kidneys cleared up."

—Sharon B.

Source: Thymic Extract: Hidden Hope to Good Health? a series of investigative reports for WAGA-FOX 5 in Atlanta, Georgia, by Michael J. Rosen, M.D.

What's in Burgstiner's Thymic Formula?

- Thymus enzymatic polypeptide fractions (containing thymosin, thymopoietin, and Thymic Humoral Factor)
- Spray/freeze-dried raw glandular extracts (including spleen, lymph, bone marrow, and pituitary extracts)
- A complete vitamin and mineral complex (including vitamins A,C,D,E, B-complex, and 10 trace and essential minerals)
- A synergistic blend of herbs, phytonutrients, amino acids, and digestive enzymes (including echinacea, bromelain, inositol, and bioflavonoids)
- Whole-food extracts (including alfalfa leaf, wheat germ, apple pectin, acidophilus, and kelp)

Action:
- Provides nutritional support for the natural synthesis of immune factors

Benefits:
- Stimulates malfunctioning immune systems
- Treats a wide variety of immune-related conditions
- Faster recovery from surgery
- Increased energy levels
- Lowers infection rates

14

SHARK-CARTILAGE THERAPY: HELP YOUR BODY CREATE NEW CARTILAGE

You have probably been led to believe that arthritis is a disease of the joints, that it is an inevitable part of the aging process, that there is fundamentally no cure. Don't believe it. Alternative doctors and researchers associated with the Health Sciences Institute have identified several underlying causes-causes your doctor may not even know to look for-that may be the source of much, if not all, of your arthritis pain. Although healing is a gradual process, pain relief can be immediate.

America's No. 1 Crippling Disease

According to the Arthritis Foundation, 40 million Americans suffer from arthritis. That's one out of every seven people of all ages. By the time you reach 60, your chances of having arthritis are close to 100 percent. In fact, arthritis is one of the most prevalent chronic health problems and the No.1 cause of limitation of movement in the United States. When you consider these statistics, it might appear to be an inevitable part of aging.

If you've tried conventional medicine, you know the truth: Drug therapy doesn't free you from pain and doesn't help to slow down your disease. What you may not know is that all conventional arthritis drugs (from NSAIDs (nonsteroidal anti-inflammatories) to steroids (carry serious risks to your health, both immediate and long-term.

The good news is that you no longer have to settle for conventional therapy. We've learned about a revolutionary treatment for joint care that relieves pain, can be used safely over the long term, and may actually help prevent joint problems.

Research suggests that it not only relieves pain and restores flexibility but may actually help cartilage regrow—something that, until now was believed impossible! This is no small feat. Unlike your liver or your heart, which can recover from devastating trauma, cartilage cannot heal itself. Once it's gone—it's gone (or so we thought).

A warning to all men and women over 35: You are losing your cartilage, little by little

Over time, the cartilage between your joints wears thin. Most doctors consider this wear and tear normal and inevitable. By the time you turn 35, you can be sure some measurable change in the shape of your cartilage has occurred. Almost everyone suffers from degenerative changes by that age. If you're over 55, your doctor probably expects to discover at least some symptoms of osteoarthritis.

There are two kinds of arthritis: you do NOT have to suffer from either

Rheumatoid arthritis is a chronic, inflammatory disorder that causes stiffness, deformity, and pain in joints and muscles (usually those of hands and feet, particularly the knuckle and toe joints.) Your joints gradually become inflamed and swollen, leading to the destruction of tissue and, in severe cases, deformity.

Unlike osteoarthritis, which progresses steadily over time, rheumatoid arthritis is a waxing/waning condition. You could have a single attack, or you might suffer several episodes that could leave you increasingly disabled. Rheumatoid arthritis is also associated with damage to the lungs, heart, nerves, and eyes. It's seen mostly in those between the ages of 40 and 60, but it can also affect children and teenagers. Three times more women than men are afflicted. The causes are not fully understood, but it's considered an autoimmune problem: Immune-system defenders attack the joint tissues as if they were threats to your body.

Osteoarthritis is very different. It's the gradual wearing away of cartilage in your joints, generally considered a process of aging. As cartilage wears thin, your joint mobility decreases. Eventually, cartilage wears through completely. Whenever you flex your joints, your bones rub against one another, causing inflammation of the synovial tissues, which cushion the joints. Movement becomes difficult and painful.

The cause? If you ask mainstream doctors, most will tell you the cause is unknown. That's the traditional stance of the Arthritis Foundation and the orthodox medical community. The standard solution? Drugs: over-the-counter pain relievers, anti-inflammatory drugs, NSAIDs, cortisone-type drugs (steroids), gold salts, and even experimental cytotoxic (cell-killing) drugs.

NSAIDs are by far the most common therapy for arthritis. If you use NSAIDs, such as ibuprofen (Motrin), naproxen (Naprosyn), oxaprozin (Daypro), nabumetone (Relafen), or diclofenac (Voltaren), you should be aware that every year almost 25,000 people using these drugs suffer serious gastrointestinal side effects, including bleeding, ulceration, and perforation.

NSAIDs also interact with blood-pressure medicine. New evidence shows their long-term use can cause liver and kidney damage. They also may accelerate the destructive nature of arthritis. These effects can occur at any time, with or without warning symptoms. Your risk increases with longer use or higher dosages.

Then there are steroids (powerful drugs that present a host of serious health risks.) To quote former Orioles baseball pitcher Jim Palmer, "Cortisone is a miracle drug...for a week!" By suppressing your immune-system response, steroids lessen swelling, soreness, and allergic reactions. In some cases, they give your body a chance to heal itself, but in the case of arthritis, they provide little more than a temporary fix.

WARNING: Steroids are strong medicines and can have very serious side effects. Since they suppress your immune system, they can lower your resistance to infections and make them harder to treat. Steroids are broad-spectrum, which means they scatter their immune-suppressing effects throughout your body(from your liver to your central nervous system. Side effects of short-term use include frequent urination, mental depression, and sudden blindness. Side effects from long-term use can include insomnia, an increase in hair growth on the body and face, an irregular heartbeat, shortness of breath, and sudden death.

Even with all of these risks, neither NSAIDs nor steroids alter the arthritis process itself. And if they don't work, surgery is usually the final option: removal of badly inflamed joint synovia, joint realignment and reconstruction, tendon repair, joint fusion, or artificial joint replacement.

Rebuilding cartilage

Yes, it is possible to rebuild cartilage. When HSI first made this statement to its members two years ago, it wasn't just controversial, it was unthinkable. Two years later, with the well-documented successes of cartilage-building substances like glucosamine and chondroitin, HSI's "audacious" assertion is now generally accepted in alternative-medicine circles.

But there's still more to the story. Glucosamine-based products fill the shelves at drugstores and health-food stores, but there are newer cartilage-regenerating products not yet on the market that promise to be even more effective than the first generation of glucosamine products. We've uncovered a breakthrough product that has not yet been publicized or widely marketed, but that you should know about immediately.

Actions:
- Acts as an anti-inflammatory
- Acts as an antiantiogenic
- Inhibits enzymes that destroy cartilage-cell proteins
- Depletes "substance P," a chemical messenger in nerve cells that transmits pain signals

Benefits:
- Delivers a natural source of glucosamine, chondroitin, and collagen directly to the joints in forms the body can more easily assimilate
- Prevents additional blood-vessel invasion of the joints in rheumatoid arthritis
- Improves the body's ability to rebuild cartilage
- Increases natural lubrication of the joints
- Reduces joint pain and inflammation
- Reduces synovitis, an inflammation of the lining of the joints

Relief from cartilage damage

Glucosamine is a nutrient found in very small amounts in food; it is also made by the cartilage cells of your body. Glucosamine plays an integral role in stimulating the production of connective tissue and new cartilage growth essential to the repair of arthritis damage. Chondroitin is another major cartilage builder and is found in bovine, shark, and whale cartilage.

As glucosamine and chondroitin formulas began filtering onto store shelves, researchers at Lane Laboratories began wondering. You see, Lane processes an ingestible form of shark cartilage, called BeneFin, that contains naturally occurring glucosamine and chondroitin and has been used successfully in the treatment of certain types of cancer for years.

When scientists at Lane studied the research findings on glucosamine and chondroitin in the treatment of arthritis, they began to wonder if shark cartilage might benefit arthritis sufferers in a way that the chemically processed versions could not. Their rationale was a simple one: If arthritis sufferers respond somewhat to glucosamine and chondroitin, would they receive an even greater benefit from the substances as they occur in nature, in the form of shark cartilage?

HSI panelist Dr. Martin Milner uses BeneFin shark cartilage extensively as a natural cancer therapy and has noted its dramatic effect on the arthritis symptoms of his patients. According to Dr. Milner, shark cartilage offers effective, naturally occurring constituents not provided by glucosamine or chondroitin supplements alone, including the following:

- Angiogenic-inhibiting proteins, substances that prevent additional blood-vessel invasion of the joints in rheumatoid arthritis (Chondroitin and glucosamine have no known effect on rheumatoid arthritis.)
- Naturally occurring glucosamine and chondroitin for the treatment of osteoarthritis, forms your body can more easily assimilate
- Collagen, which has a body of evidence supporting its efficacy in treating arthritis
- Calcium and phosphorus (15% and 7% respectively by weight), both of which are important for maintaining bone health and recommended by the FDA to fight osteoporosis

A more efficient delivery system

Recently, shark-cartilage therapy has made an exciting new advance. Typically, shark cartilage is administered orally, in a powdered form. However, it appears that shark cartilage can also be absorbed directly through the skin, delivering the substance directly to the desired location, with all of its constituents intact and with a minimum of fuss.

Apply it directly to your joints

Lane Labs has extended this line of research to the creation of an odorless shark cartilage cream designed especially for the targeted treatment of arthritis pain and inflammation. The new product is called BeneJoint, and it is unique among topical arthritis creams. It combines the restorative power of shark cartilage with the pain-relieving compound capsaicin.

Capsaicin is a natural substance derived from cayenne pepper. It works by depleting "substance P," a chemical messenger in nerve cells that transmits pain signals. BeneJoint is the only product that combines the analgesic action of capsaicin with the cartilage-building substances in shark cartilage.

"I've had arthritis in my lumbar spine for a couple of years. I had X-rays taken, and I went to a specialist who told me I have a lot of spurs. The pain gets worse all the time. I tried Mineral Ice, but it really never helped much. I've done exercises—you name it, I've tried it. I work for Lane Labs, and people there asked if I would like to try a sample of BeneJoint for my arthritis. After only three or four days, it was really helping me—I could bend down without feeling pain! I was so impressed with the product that I told many of my mother's friends who have arthritis about it, and they're anxious to try it too. I'm hoping this will help a lot of people."

—Regina F., Fairlawn, NJ

Because BeneJoint delivers a natural source of glucosamine and chondroitin directly to the joints, this cream may be used in conjunction with other nutrient-based arthritis therapies for maximal benefit. See page 152 for sources.

15

IPRIFLAVONE:
PREVENT AND REVERSE OSTEOPOROSIS

STUDIES SHOW INCREASED BONE MASS, REDUCED FRACTURES, AND DECREASE IN PAIN

The multiple benefits of soy are well-documented. Natural chemicals found in soy—such as gensitein, isoflavones, saponins, and phytosterols—have been shown to protect against many types of cancer, prevent coronary artery disease, boost the immune system, and relieve symptoms of menopause.

Now, however, a newly identified soy isolate called ipriflavone offers a potent weapon for the millions of people threatened by, or already suffering from, osteoporosis.

In the short time since the discovery of ipriflavone, over 60 human clinical studies in Europe and Japan have already proven that it is readily absorbed in the body and reduces bone loss, bone pain, loss of mobility, and vertebral fractures in osteoporotic patients.[1] These same studies have demonstrated supplemental ipriflavone to be completely safe and without any major side effects.

- In one clinical study, postmenopausal women given ipriflavone combined with vitamin D showed a significant reduction in vertebral bone loss.[2]
- Another study confirmed ipriflavone's inability to elicit estrogenic activity on other organs. This is important, since ipriflavone exerts the bone-building properties of estrogen without the estrogenic effects on other organ systems.[3]
- A study performed at the University of Budapest shows that ipriflavone can reverse bone damage and reduce pain and suffering. Patients in this study actually increased lost bone mass, while enjoying reduced pain and increased mobility.[4]

---
[1] *Calcified Tissue International*, vol. 61, no. 2, pp. 142-147, 1997
[2] *International Journal of Gynecology & Obstetrics*, vol. 48, pp. 283-288, 1995
[3] *Journal of Endocrinology Investigation*, vol. 15, pp. 755-761, 1992
[4] *Acta Pharmacology Hungary*, vol. 65, no. 6, pp. 229-232, 1995

- A study at the University of Bologna in Italy shows that women on hormone-replacement therapy who add ipriflavone enjoy a significant boost in bone density compared to taking hormone-replacement therapy alone.[5]

What if I'm sensitive to soy?

Although a diet high in soy-based foods like tofu, miso, and tempeh offers many health benefits, many people cannot readily digest whole soy. For them, soy can cause painful gas, bloating, and abdominal discomfort. Soy is also one of the most frequent culprits in delayed food sensitivities. If you're not digesting it well, you certainly can't reap the health benefits soy has to offer.

Once ipriflavone is isolated from whole soy, however, it no longer contains the soy proteins that cause the digestive difficulties associated with soy-based foods. So even those with soy sensitivities can benefit from the bone-saving powers of ipriflavone therapy.

Estrogen: not a panacea

Although you may know that estrogen is often used to prevent osteoporosis, you may not be aware that the amount needed to reduce the incidence of osteoporosis is sufficient to cause serious side effects, including excessive bleeding, breast pain, and an increased risk of breast and ovarian cancers.

What about "low-dose" estrogen therapy? Low-dose estrogen may ward off hot flashes and other hormone-associated symptoms, but the low dosage is not significant enough to prevent osteoporosis. Yet estrogen continues to be the most frequently prescribed medication in America.

The latest osteoporosis drug...it's the same old story

You may also have heard about raloxifene, a potent drug-with substantial side effects-being heralded in the treatment of osteoporosis. While it appears to be effective in helping to prevent osteoporosis, the drug (trade name Evista) increases one's chances of serious blood-clot formation. It also brings back menstrual periods in postmenopausal women. Worse yet, the FDA panel approving the drug noted that "two-year studies are not long enough to be sure a breast-cancer risk would never appear."

---

[1] *Osteoporosis International*, vol. 5, no. 6, pp. 462-466, 1995

The multiple myths of osteoporosis

MYTH NO. 1

Osteoporosis is an old person's disease.

If you believe (as many do) that osteoporosis is something to be concerned about after middle age, you need to know that it actually begins in your 20s, when your body becomes less efficient at absorbing minerals from food. As a result, the body often begins to "borrow" these minerals from bone stores. Eventually, the bones become brittle, weak, and prone to fracture.

MYTH NO. 2

Osteoporosis affects women only.

While being a woman increases your risk of developing osteoporosis, the disease is not limited to women. The truth is that one in eight men over 50 will break a bone due to osteoporosis. And a broken hip is more likely to lead to death in men than in women.

MYTH NO. 3

Calcium will keep your bones strong.

While calcium can be effective in helping to prevent osteoporosis, it alone is not enough. Other minerals are necessary to promote its effective use by your body. For example, you need magnesium, too, in a ratio of 2:1 of calcium over magnesium, in order for your body to effectively utilize the calcium.

According to leading nutritionist Carl Germano, author of *The Osteoporosis Solution*, "Bone is living tissue that contains much more than just the hard material we picture as bone. Calcium does nothing about the spongy, soft aspect of bone that keeps us flexible without breaking. Vitamin D, manganese, and boron, for example, are also crucial to the process of forming and maintaining healthy bones."

THE FACTS:

Every year, 700,000 people suffer spinal fractures due to osteoporosis.

This year alone, 300,000 people will break a hip because of osteoporosis, and 20 percent of them will die within a year of the fracture.

Putting ipriflavone to work for you

With the use of natural bone-protecting nutrients like ipriflavone, much of the pain and trauma of osteoporosis can be avoided and unnecessary deaths prevented. It may be years before mainstream medicine recognizes this important advance, but that doesn't mean you have to wait to safeguard your bone health naturally.

Since the research supporting the use of supplementary ipriflavone to prevent and treat osteoporosis is brand-new in this country, we were hard-pressed to locate a source. We did find one new product called OsteoSupport that combines ipriflavone with isoflavones, calcium, and magnesium in optimal proportions, as well as with other nutrients designed to work together to promote optimal bone health. OsteoSupport can be ordered from the source listed on page 149.

Action:
- Exerts the bone-building properties of estrogen without having estrogenic effects on other organ systems

Benefits:
- Reverses bone loss
- Reverses bone damage
- Reduces pain
- Reduces loss of mobility
- Reduces vertebral fractures in osteoporotic patients
- Increases bone density

16

RA Spes: Ancient Asia Formula Controls Rheumatoid Arthritis

Patients Report Profound Relief After Just Two Weeks

Paulette R.'s rheumatoid arthritis is severe. The pain sometimes gets so intense that she is unable to turn over in bed. Her doctors prescribed steroids to control the inflammation in her joints and narcotics for the pain. The drugs help, but not enough.

Recently, however, Paulette was given a natural herbal product called RA Spes. Her experience with RA Spes has been so remarkable that Paulette is anxious to get the word out to fellow rheumatoid-arthritis sufferers:

"I tell everyone with rheumatoid arthritis that they should be on it. I have completely weaned myself off of Prednisone and am only taking RA Spes. It is such a relief to be able to stop taking the steroids—I was very concerned about the long-term effects. And RA Spes is controlling my arthritis much better than the drugs did.

"I ran out last month, and after two or three days the pain was so intense that I could not dress myself or move. My husband had to help me with everything...including feeding me. Just eight hours after I started again on the RA Spes, I got relief.

"Thank you for RA Spes. Please don't ever let this product run out. Without it, life is awful."

"Spes" is the Latin word for "hope". If you suffer from rheumatoid arthritis, RA Spes offers new hope for a more comfortable, active, and independent life.

We still don't know what causes the body to destroy its own joints

Rheumatoid arthritis (RA) is a relentless and crippling form of arthritis that affects about one out of every 100 people. It is generally considered an autoimmune disorder, in which the immune cells mistakenly target the body's own tissue—in this case, the synovial tissue that surrounds your joints. But the primary cause of rheumatoid arthritis is not yet fully understood. Leading researchers are investigating the possibility that infectious agents, such as viruses or bacteria, may trigger the disease.

RA is characterized by pain, inflammation, and the gradual deterioration of the cartilage and bone tissue in the joints (especially the fingers, wrists, elbows, shoulders, spine, hips, and knees). In severe cases, RA can invade the organs of the body, affecting the eyes, heart, lungs, and nerves. In one out of 10 cases, the damage is so devastating that the patient is eventually confined to a bed or wheelchair.

Conventional medicine has no cure

Women are two or three times more likely than men to have RA, but if anyone in your immediate family suffers from it, your risk is increased. Conventional medicine has no cure, it focuses mainly on relieving pain and inflammation with NSAIDs and/or steroids.

Steroids are effective but extremely dangerous. By comparison, NSAIDs may seem pretty harmless. But a steady diet of ibuprofen can lead to stomach bleeding, liver toxicity, or worse. (In fact, iron-deficiency anemia is common in arthritis sufferers. Constant use of NSAIDS can lead to low-grade gastrointestinal blood loss, depleting the body's iron stores.)

In more severe cases, doctors often try antirheumatic drugs (DMARDs), which aim to slow the progression of the disease. DMARDs do nothing for the pain, however, and the side effects are so severe that the majority of patients opt to stop taking them, even when they are working. As a final resort, mainstream practitioners prescribe surgery to remove swollen joint tissue or completely replace ruined joints.

It's no wonder so many arthritis sufferers turn in desperation to alternative medicine for answers.

Seeking botanical solutions

If you've shopped in health-food stores for natural arthritis remedies, you're probably familiar with the anti-inflammatory botanicals. They include ginger, turmeric (found in curry powder), bromelain (from pineapple), boswellia, and others. They are used for all kinds of arthritis and other inflammatory conditions.

However, these still only address one symptom of arthritis—

inflammation—and not the cause. Because RA is a progressive disease, a real and lasting solution must go beyond symptomatic relief and succeed in slowing or reversing the disease process itself. For this, you must approach the disease at its foundation: your immune system.

An ancient formula of Chinese herbs targets RA at its source

One of our contacts led us to RA Spes—the product that made such a dramatic difference for Paulette. RA Spes is a unique herbal remedy based on a traditional Chinese formula for rheumatic conditions. It goes far beyond symptomatic relief—it actually helps to correct the immunological malfunctions that cause RA to develop and progress.

Unless you are a student of traditional Chinese medicine, many of the herbs used in RA Spes may be unfamiliar to you. Below are the ingredients (listed by both their Chinese and Latin names):

Wu-chia-pi (Acanthopanax senticosus Harms)
Tse-hsieh (Alisma plantago-aquatica L.)
Ai-yeh (Artemisia capillaris T.)
Chai-hu (Bupleurum Chinense DC)
Yen-hu-suo (Corydalis bulbosa)
Shan-yao (Dioscorea opposita T.)
Gan-cao (Glycyrrhiza glabra L.)
Wu-wei-zi (Schizandra chinensis Baill)
Huang-chin (Scutellaria baicalensis)

According to traditional Chinese medicine, these herbs promote blood circulation, clear pathogenic heat and toxins, expel dampness, strengthen vital energy, and balance the Qi energy of the kidney.

Modern research has verified that these herbs also reduce inflammation, relieve pain, cleanse the liver, invigorate circulation, and tone the organs of the elimination system, including the skin, kidneys, and bowels.

And now, recent clinical trials, published in the *Chinese Journal of Rheumatic Disease*,1 have found that, in addition to relieving pain and reducing joint swelling, RA Spes is a potent immune modulator, actually slowing the progress of the disease.

After only two weeks on RA Spes, the subjects' blood tests showed dramatic improvement in seven different immunological markers of rheumatoid arthritis. In comparison, steroids and NSAIDs had no positive immunological effect at all and in some cases actually reduced immune function.

What does this mean for your quality of life?

Blood markers like HLA-DR+ cell counts and B-lymphocyte proliferation rates may be exciting to researchers, but what does all this mean to you? In addition to looking at the lab tests and blood work, researchers also evaluated each patient's quality of life and symptoms like stiffness, swelling, and joint pain. The results were striking:

- Clinical symptoms (pain, swelling, and stiffness) were reduced by 50 percent after the first two weeks. After three months, the symptoms were reduced by almost 90 percent.
- Quality of life was dramatically upgraded after three months. Patients who had been previously confined to a bed or wheelchair were able to move around independently. The most significant improvements were noted in the more severe cases.
- Using standardized evaluation criteria developed by the American College of Rheumatology, patients using RA Spes improved by 80 percent after two weeks and by 90 percent after one month.

Most patients took four to six capsules a day. No serious side effects were reported. Even better, because the subjects stopped taking other drugs during the trial, many enjoyed relief from unpleasant side effects of their previous medication.

Due to the costs involved in procuring and processing the Chinese herbs, the price of RA Spes is somewhat high—from $100 to $400 a month, depending on the dosage (a bottle of 30 capsules costs $60).

But as Paulette put it, "How can you put a price on getting your life back? I feel so much better now that I'm off the drugs. After only three weeks on RA Spes, my energy has increased tenfold. I had forgotten what it was like to feel this good!"

HSI panelist Dr. Robert Yee has over 20 years' experience in integrating Eastern and Western medical approaches. He is very impressed with the science and theory behind RA Spes: "In Chinese medicine, herbs are used not only for their biochemical actions. They are also intended to affect the energy patterns of certain diseases—to balance the various systems of the body and correct the flow of Qi, or energy. And, of course, laboratory tests cannot yet measure the energetic dimension of these herbs.

"But there's no doubt that this botanical formula is effective—both chemically and energetically. RA Spes is a very valuable product—I would

---

[1] *Chinese Journal of Rheumatic Disease Based on Integrated Traditional and Western Medicine*, vol. 3, no. 3, pp. 29-33, 1985

not hesitate to recommend it to patients with rheumatoid arthritis."

You can order RA Spes from the source listed on page 152.

Actions:
- Contains a powerful immune-system modulator
- Promotes blood circulation
- Acts as an Anti-inflammatory
- Cleanses the liver
- Tones the organs of the elimination system.

Benefits:
- Slows the progress of rheumatoid arthritis in addition to relieving joint pain and swelling
- No unpleasant side effects

17

LARREASTAT: RELIEF FOR VICTIMS OF HERPES AND RHEUMATOID ARTHRITIS

In one of the most exciting developments of the decade, researchers recently released their findings on a new, natural product that has been shown to be 99.7 percent effective in the relief of symptoms brought on by the herpes viruses.

If you think that this good news applies only to a few, you may be surprised to learn that, according to recent estimates, up to 99 percent of the population may be infected with one or more of the many herpes viruses. (The most well-known is the virus that causes chicken pox.) These viruses can lie dormant for years before exhibiting any symptoms, and unsuspecting carriers can easily infect others.

When triggered by stress, infections, or diseases like cancer, herpes viruses can manifest themselves as cold sores, genital lesions, chicken pox, and shingles. Various strains have also been linked to mononucleosis, chronic fatigue syndrome, and Kaposi's sarcoma, a deadly type of skin cancer frequently, but not exclusively, affecting people with AIDS.

In addition, there is a growing body of evidence that a herpes virus called cytomegalovirus (CMV) plays a causal role in cardiovascular disease.

About 75 percent of Americans over 60 carry CMV, with no observable symptoms. But if the virus is "turned on," it appears to play a role in the clogging of artery walls.[1] Possible triggers include balloon angioplasty and heart-transplant surgery.

And in another startling development, scientists have linked the Simplex I virus with Alzheimer's disease.[2] Apparently, the Simplex I virus can lodge in brain tissue and replicate at a very low level. Although the replication is too subtle to cause acute disease symptoms, it is enough to activate the immune system. It is possible that the

---

[1] Nieto Javier, et. al., "CMV infection as a risk factor for carotid intimal-medial thickening," Circulation, vol. 94, no. 5, 1996, pp. 922-7;S.E. Epstein, et. al., "The role of infection in restenosis and atherosclerosis," Lancet, vol. 348, Suppl. 1, 1996, pp. 13-17.
[2] Andrew Chavallier, The Encylopedia of Medicinal Plants, vol. 21, 1997, p. 224.

resulting inflammatory reaction, over years, may eventually lead to Alzheimer's disease.

And so it was for good reason that researchers in Arizona were elated at the results of studies, confirmed by independent clinical tests, showing that a new "botaniceutical" product derived from the Larrea bush could cripple these insidious viruses without side effects of any kind. By contrast, side effects of acyclovir (Zorivax), the drug commonly prescribed to manage herpes symptoms, include headaches, seizures, coma, nausea, vomiting, and diarrhea. More importantly, prolonged or repeated use of acyclovir can actually encourage the proliferation of drug-resistant strains of the herpes virus.

An ancient desert bush yields this remarkable healing agent

This new preparation is made from an ancient desert bush, Larrea tridentata, used medicinally for centuries by Native Americans as well as early European settlers of the southwestern United States. According to Native American legend, it was the first plant created at the beginning of the world. Scientists have in fact validated that these shrubs are among the oldest living plants on earth, some plants dating back to over 12,000 years ago.

Traditionally, Larrea was used to treat infections, snakebite, burns, rheumatism, bronchitis, colds and viruses, and digestive disorders. The phenomenon of an all-purpose natural panacea is not a new one to Health Sciences Institute members. A wide range of effective applications is the hallmark of a natural remedy. These do not work through a single, isolated action, as do our modern pharmaceuticals, but through the varied and synergistic actions of myriad phytochemical compounds.

Clearly, the Larrea shrub, also known in the Southwest as the creosote bush and to herbalists as chaparral, is a potent natural healer. Listed in the Pharmacopoeia of the United States from 1842 to 1942, chaparral was widely used to treat acne, eczema, venereal and urinary infections, and even certain types of cancer, particularly leukemia.2 In the 1960s, promising research on the antitumor properties of one of chapparal's chief constituents was abandoned when long-term use in lab animals suggested toxicity.[3] In the early 1990s, a few cases of hepatitis were tied to use of the herb and the FDA requested a voluntary ban on products containing raw chapparal. (Scientists later determined the cases

---

[3] Varro Tyler, Ph.D., The Honest Herbal, 1993, p. 87.

to be unrelated to chapparal use.)[4]

As we have noted before, the fact that something is natural does not mean that it is necessarily harmless. Herbs can be extremely potent, as any student of herbal medicine can attest, and it is possible for an herb to have a toxic effect. Nonetheless, one group of scientists refused to abandon the healing potential of chaparral and continued to search for a way to isolate the beneficial properties of the Larrea bush.

After a decade of research, it appears they have succeeded. Researchers identified a matrix of natural chemicals that appear to be responsible for Larrea's medicinal qualities. Through a proprietary process, they have purified, concentrated, and solubilized these phytochemicals, documented their biological activity, and thoroughly tested them for toxicity of any kind. The oxidative components of the raw plant believed to be responsible for any toxicity have been eliminated. The result is a natural product that exploits all of the healing potential attributed for centuries to this desert shrub but, according to extensive testing, is safe. Even at doses five times the equivalent human dose, test animals remained in excellent health. Enzyme studies on liver and kidney functions showed no ill effects.

The herpes/rheumatoid-arthritis connection

Many herpes viruses hide out in nerve tissue. People who have shingles often feel a burning pain in their nerves before the shingles appear. This is because the zoster virus that causes shingles starts replicating in the nerves before it actually breaks through to the skin.

But researchers have recently learned that a certain group of herpes viruses can hide in the connective tissue. This group of viruses, called the gamma-herpes viruses, includes Epstein-Barr and HHV-8. It is theorized that these gamma viruses may be a hidden cause of rheumatoid arthritis and other connective tissue disorders.

The good news about rheumatoid-arthritis relief

Although the remarkable results of this new product for herpes sufferers are stealing the headlines, there have been equally dramatic reports of relief for rheumatoid-arthritis sufferers. An 18-year-old patient suffering from juvenile rheumatoid arthritis for seven years got only minimum relief from even high doses of prescription anti-

---

[4] Michael Castleman, "Herbal Healthwatch," Herb Quarterly, Spring 1996, p. 6

inflammatories. Upon rising in the morning, the patient was so stiff that he could not walk down the stairs. After using Larreastat capsules for only two weeks, this young man is now playing basketball and holding a full-time summer job.

A 70-year-old California woman with chronic rheumatoid arthritis and long-standing pain and immobility in her knee joint reported over 90 percent relief from pain and swelling and could walk normally again after using Larreastat capsules for two weeks. Numerous other patients of collaborating physicians report dramatic improvements.

How can this preparation be so effective for such seemingly unrelated conditions as herpes and rheumatoid arthritis? For the same reason that the Larrea plant has been used successfully for centuries for a wide range of conditions. Larrea is rich in a powerful antioxidant lignan called nordihydroguaiaretic acid (NDGA), as well as several other chemically related lignans. Lignans are phytochemicals that show significant antioxidant, anti-inflammatory, antiviral, and antimicrobial properties. In fact, before the modern food industry developed cheaper, synthetic preservatives, NDGA was widely used as a food preservative. It prevents the oxidation of fats and oils in foods, thereby inhibiting the growth of a wide variety of bacteria, yeast, and fungi.

Clearly, Larrea's strong antiviral action makes it a useful weapon against the herpes viruses. But NDGA has also been shown to inhibit 5-lipoxygenase, an enzyme involved in the biochemical process known as the inflammatory cascade. This suggests why Larrea has such a dramatic impact on the symptoms of rheumatoid arthritis, a chronic inflammation caused by the overactivity of the inflammatory cascade in the body.

Furthermore, Larrea is a source of over two dozen flavonoid compounds, many of which are not found in any other known dietary source. These chemicals, which work synergistically with other antioxidant vitamins, especially vitamin C, provide further antioxidant, anti-inflammatory, and antiviral properties. Flavonoids also work to strengthen capillaries, enhancing the transport of nutrients to the tissues of the body.

Because Larreastat products have shown such remarkable ability against diseases for which there are currently so few effective treatments, they represent an important new botanaceutical development. See the "Guide to Sources and Availability," page 150.

Actions:
- Inhibits a critical enzyme in the inflammation process
- Prevents oxidative damage
- Strengthens capillaries

Benefits:
- Alleviates pain and inflammation
- Inhibits the growth of viruses, bacteria, yeast, and fungi
- Enhances the transport of nutrients

Dramatic Relief from Herpes Symptoms

The new Larrea product is formulated both as a topical lotion that can be applied directly to herpes lesions and as a nutritional supplement that can be used to help avert impending outbreaks or to speed healing. Here are only a few of the dozens of successful outcomes confirmed in recent clinical trials:

- A woman suffering from recurrent oral herpes previously used acyclovir with only mixed results. After a single application of the Larrea preparation, lesions were completely healed in 12 hours. Pain and swelling were relieved immediately.
- A 90-year-old woman had Kaposi's sarcoma lesions that covered her body from head to toe. Lesions on her lower extremities were so advanced that one toe had already been amputated. Acyclovir was used without success.

After three weeks of treatment twice daily with Larreastat lotion, the lesions on her arm, face, and feet had completely cleared.

- A clinic in Philadelphia treated numerous patients with severe herpes simplex 1 and 2 and zoster (shingles) with both the Larreastat lotion and capsules. They report a 100 percent success rate, usually within 24-48 hours. The clinicians also report success using the lotion to avert impending outbreaks, which are usually signaled by a tingling sensation.
- A woman with oral herpes typically had outbreaks lasting three to seven days. When she applied the lotion to a new blister, the pain, swelling, and blistering were gone in one day.

- Shingles sufferers who were treated with Larreastat reported complete relief within minutes.

In dozens of case histories reviewed, one phrase appeared repeatedly: "complete resolution of the episode within 24 hours." No side effects were reported by any subjects.

SECTION V
Brain Power and Mental Health

Now there's no need to fear the loss of your cognitive abilities as you age—in this section of Underground Cures 1999, you'll read about amazing brain boosters like DHA and phosphatidylserine. These substances fight the effects of Alzheimer's Disease and the "mental decline" that can come with aging, such as trouble concentrating, a tendency to forget things, prolonged depression, and difficulty in recalling newly learned information. See also the chapter on Cardiocysteine Formula (page 53) for more information on battling the effects of Alzheimer's Disease.

Also in this section, we discuss the natural alternatives to commonly prescribed antidepressants like Prozac and Zoloft: These natural products can do a great deal for your well being without addictive qualities and potentially dangerous side effects. Organic germanium is also effective for improving mood and energy level. You can read about organic germanium in the your heart-health section on page 63.

18

PHOSPHATIDYLSERINE—
THE ONE TRUE SMART PILL

Can't remember where you put the car keys? Having trouble absorbing new information—even if it's as simple as a phone number or an appointment? Can't remember if you've already "told that story before?"

Symptoms of "mental decline"—which include trouble concentrating, a tendency to forget things, prolonged depression, and difficulty in recalling newly learned information—start as early as age 50 and become pronounced and outwardly

As frightening, embarrassing, and frustrating as these symptoms are, it's no wonder the hot new item on the alternative-medicine market these days is the "smart pill." Walk into any health-food store, and you'll find dozens of herbal brain-health supplement programs. These formulas are almost guaranteed to contain significant amounts of herbs like ginseng, which has demonstrated the ability to improve endurance- and Ginkgo biloba, which has the unparalleled ability to fight peripheral vascular disease. Ginkgo not only frees up blood flow to the brain but also protects your delicate brain cells from free-radical damage.

Both herbs are well-established in the alternative-medicine community as treatments for depression and all-around 'mental fog.' In Europe, Ginkgo biloba is routinely prescribed in a standardized, concentrated form to help the elderly reverse many conditions related to problems of circulation, such as tinnitus (ringing in the ears), confusion, dizziness, headaches, and memory loss.

Both of these exceptional herbs have been proven in hundreds of cultures around the world, in study after study, to have significant brain-enhancing benefits.

But the one thing these products CANNOT do is improve your actual brain mechanisms: the delicate cellular relationships that are responsible for everything from recognition and recall to mood and outlook.

In other words, these popular smart pills may enhance the circulation to your brain or augment your mood-regulating hormones, but they simply do not improve the function of the brain itself. Such a substance would truly be a miracle—real-life smart pill.

Can you improve the inner workings of your brain? In a word, yes.

There is a naturally derived substance that can literally prevent and reverse the "normal" mental decline that comes with age. It can in fact, do all of the following:

- boost your ability to learn
- improve your ability to remember NEW information
- improve your visual memory
- improve your memorization skills

According to some researchers, this powerful nutrient may be able to reverse more than a decade's worth of mental decline!

It's called phosphatidylserine (PS). PS—an essential fatty acid your body produces naturally in limited amounts—keeps your brain active and alert, starting on the cellular level.

First, it "influences fluidity" of the brain-cell membrane. By facilitating the delivery of nutrients to the brain cells, as well as the cells' ability to receive the nutrients, PS effectively feeds your brain.

Second, it activates the nerve cells and nerve-transmitter production. This means it helps regulate and stimulate the instantaneous "flashes" of information and your ability to react to that information. It even gives you more brain circuits with which to communicate by actually increasing the number of neurotransmitter receptor sites.

Third, as shown in tests with rats, PS blocks the decline of nerve growth factor, which seems to occur naturally as we age.

Fourth, PS has been shown to have antioxidant properties, which means it protects your brain cells from the damage done by free radicals.

Of all the organs in your body, your brain is the most vulnerable to attack by free radicals. Free radicals are the nasty, ravenous molecules that eat away—literally—at the core of your good health. Like an apple that turns brown and rots in the open air—so the delicate tissues of your vital organs decay—ravaged by free radicals oxidizing your cells.

Simply put, PS protects and RENEWS your brain—at any age

Although your body does produce PS in limited amounts, as you age, you produce less and less. If you want to keep your brain functioning optimally, it is critical that you replenish your levels of PS regularly. Though certain foods contain this critical nutrient, the concentrations are not high enough to raise your PS levels. The best way to replenish your PS stores is through daily supplementation.

How to go back in time 12 "brain-age" years

When you replenish your PS levels, you not only boost your brain power-you may actually reverse your brain age!

Just consider the results of one study of 149 people, age 50 or older, who had "normal" age-related memory loss. Some study participants took 100 mg of PS three times a day for 12 weeks; the others, unknown to them, took placebos. By the end of the experiment, the people taking PS benefited from a 15 percent improvement in learning and other memory tasks, with the greatest benefit coming to those with the greatest impairment. Plus, these significant benefits continued for up to four weeks after stopping PS.

Clinical psychologist Thomas Crook, one of the study's authors, said the study suggests that PS "may reverse approximately 12 years of decline." (*Neurology*, vol. 41, no. 5, 1991.)

In another 12-week study, 51 people (average age: 71) took PS supplements and improved their short-term memory. They could better recall names and the locations of misplaced objects. They remembered more details of recent events and could concentrate more intently. (*Psychopharmacology Bulletin*, vol. 28, 1992.)

"Vigilance and concentration"

In other studies, PS showed great promise for those with Alzheimer's disease, Parkinson's disease, and circulation diseases (arteriosclerotic cerebrovascular disease). In particular, those with cerebrovascular disease experienced improvements linked to "vigilance, concentration, and motor reaction" (Ransmayr et al., double-blind trial., 1978).

Plus, PS may also help alleviate depression (Maggioni et al., 1990, double-blind trial, 1990), as well as significantly lower the production of a stress hormone called cortisol.

PS may one day be as widely taken as vitamins C and E, as more and more researchers discover how critical it is to good mental functioning. There are many PS products on the market, and we've reviewed many of them. One we recommend is Brain Power Plus, which includes optimal amounts of the nutrients PS, Acetyl-L-carnitine, DHA, Ginkgo biloba,

Panax ginseng, and Siberian ginseng. Brain Power Plus also contains red-date extract, which is used in traditional Chinese medicine to enhance the activity of ginseng; schizandra, a powerful antioxidant that assists with mental clarity and increases your body's level of the detoxifying enzyme glutathione; and the traditional Indian "brain tonic" gotu kolu, which is used in Ayurvedic medicine to improve mental agility and reduce anxiety and depression. See the "Guide to Sources and Availability" on page 151 for the source of Brain Power Plus.

Actions:

- Activates nerve cells and neurotransmitter production
- Influences cell-membrane fluidity and facilitates delivery of nutrients to brain cells
- Blocks the decline of nerve growth factor
- Acts as an antioxidant

Benefits:

- Helps keep the brain active and alert
- Boosts your ability to learn information
- Improves visual memory
- Helps in alleviating depression

---

[1] Gindin, J. et al., "The Effect of Plant Phosphatidylserine on Age Associated Memory Impairment and Mood in the Functioning Elderly." Geriatric Institute for Education and Research and Department of Geriatrics, Kaplan Hospital, Rehovot Hospital. (1995)
[2] Mantovani, P, et al., In Function and Metabolism of Phospholipids, ed. by Porcellati G and others, New York: Plenum Press, pp. 285-92, 1976.
[3] Kidd PM, "Phosphatidylserine, membrane nutrient for memory." A clinic and mechanistic assessment. *Alternative Medicine Review*, vol. 1, no. 2, July/August.

19

DHA: BOOST YOUR BRAINPOWER

One of today's most popular heart supplements, the omega-3 fish oil docosahexaenoic acid (DHA, not to be confused with the hormone DHEA) is likely to be tomorrow's most sought-after brain pill. In Norway, doctors regularly prescribe DHA to lower cholesterol. In the United States, it's available in health-food stores and is known for its ability to greatly lower the risk of a sudden deadly heart attack. It's also well-known as an important nutrient for pregnant women, since DHA is crucial to fetal brain development.

The latest research from Japan demonstrates why DHA is also necessary to maintain optimum brain functioning in adults, and why it could turn out to be critical for the prevention and possible reversal of Alzheimer's disease!

Keeping your brain alive, active, and alert—cell by cell

You have approximately 14 billion brain cells, each of which connects and "talks" to other brain cells by sending signals through electrical "arms" called axons. This communication is the basis for learning and memory, as well as for sending messages of pain and pleasure throughout your body. When the arms between brain cells are flexible and pliant, the communication operates at its best. Studies show that DHA is critical to maintaining soft and flexible axons, thus keeping your brain healthy and active.

When the level of DHA drops, reducing axon flexibility, the arms become hardened and signals are transmitted more slowly. Researchers in Japan have recently observed that the absence of DHA is associated with many cognitive and mental-health conditions, such as depression, schizophrenia, and dementia of the Alzheimer's type.

DHA as a treatment for Alzheimer's

Early tests on treatment with DHA have been very promising. In a study performed at Gunma National University in Japan, patients suffering from symptoms of Alzheimer's disease showed a 65 percent improvement in symptoms of dementia with the use of DHA.

In another study, researchers formulated their own omega-3 oil product to make sure it had a very high concentration of DHA (53 percent), because, they write, most of the current "omega-3 fish-oil products are low in DHA content (12 percent) and are primarily marketed for heart disease." The researchers wanted to test the maximum effects of DHA on brain function, so they significantly increased the percentage of DHA and conducted a memory study with lab animals. The results of their 20-day investigation showed that (1) DHA improves memory and (2) the higher the dose, the better the results.

How to choose the best source of DHA

You have to be very particular when you're looking for your DHA supplement, because, as noted, the majority of the fish oils you'll find in the health-food stores have been prepared as heart-health supplements and are not going to give your brain the support it needs.

Look for a fish-oil supplement with a high ratio of DHA to EPA. (EPA, eicosapentaoic acid, as you may already know, lowers cholesterol, but it also has an anticlotting effect you want to avoid.) Try to find a supplement derived from tuna; of all the cold-water fish, tuna has the highest DHA content. A good ratio of DHA to EPA would be 25 to 30 percent DHA to 7 percent or less EPA.

While your body can synthesize most fats, there are a few that are considered "essential" because you must obtain them from food or supplements. DHA is an essential fatty acid. You need to continually refresh your brain's supply. And here's an extra tip for improving your brain health: One study showed that DHA was even more effective for those who eat fish at least five times a week in addition to taking the DHA.

The recommended amount for DHA supplementation is 750 milligrams a day. For purchasing information, see the "Guide to Sources and Availability" on page 148.

Actions:
- Nourishes and supports neural synapses
- Enhances synapse flexibility
- Promotes nerve-signal transmission
- Lowers cholesterol

Benefits:
- Improves memory and mental functioning
- May protect against depression, schizophrenia, and dementia (Alzheimer's disease)
- Reduces the risk of a sudden deadly heart attack

20

INOSITOL: NUTRIENT THERAPY FOR ALZHEIMER'S DISEASE, DEPRESSION, AND ANXIETY

Inositol, a lesser-known B-vitamin, has recently come into the limelight as a surprising new superstar in a variety of psychiatric and neurological disorders, including Alzheimer's disease, depression, anxiety, obsessive compulsive disorder, and panic disorder.

Inositol is commonly found in foods that contain other B vitamins, like lecithin, brewer's yeast, liver, wheat germ, and whole grains. As HSI panelist Elson Haas, M.D. explains in *Staying Healthy with Nutrition* (Celestial Arts, 1992, p. 136), "The body can produce its own inositol from glucose, so it is not really essential. We have high stores of inositol; its concentration in the body is second highest of the B vitamins, surpassed only by niacin."

With no real danger of deficiency, the importance of inositol might easily be overlooked. But recent research reveals that inositol in therapeutic amounts has led to dramatic results in a number of double-blind, placebo-controlled studies:

Alzheimer's disease. A small trial evaluated the effects of 6000 mg a day of inositol on sufferers of Alzheimer's disease. After only one month, those using inositol showed significant improvement in language and orientation, as compared to the control (placebo) group. Researchers intend to study larger doses and longer trial periods (*Neuro-psychopharm. Biological Psychiatry*, vol. 20, pp. 729-735, 1996).

Obsessive-Compulsive Disorder (OCD). Based on a six-week study, researchers concluded that inositol was effective in managing OCD and other serotonin-related disorders. Subjects taking 18 grams a day of inositol showed significant improvement in OCD symptoms. These were patients who had not responded to treatment with pharmaceutical antidepressants (selective serotonin reuptake inhibitors, or SSRIs) or had been disturbed by side effects. (*American Journal of Psychiatry*, vol. 153, pp. 1219-1221, 1996).

Panic disorder. Researchers noted a decrease in frequency and severity of panic attacks among patients using 12 grams of inositol a day for four weeks. No significant side effects were noted. (*American Journal of Psychiatry*, vol. 152, pp. 1084-1086, 1995).

Depression. Subjects taking 12 grams a day of inositol displayed significant improvement on the Hamilton Depression Rating Scale after one month, as compared to the control group. (*American Journal of Psychiatry*, vol. 152, pp. 792-794, 1995).

Inositol is found in large amounts in brain tissue and plays an important role in nerve-cell communication. One of its functions is as a "secondary messenger" or backup system for the regulation of serotonin levels in the brain. This helps to explain why therapeutic amounts of inositol appear to help those individuals whose conditions don't respond to SSRIs like Prozac. It also represents an alternative for those who suffer unpleasant side effects (such as nausea, headache, insomnia, and a reduced sex drive) from SSRIs.

A typical multivitamin formula might include only 50 mg of inositol, if it includes any at all. But the research suggests that dosages of up to 18 grams (or 18,000 mg) are indicated for some conditions. Some researchers believe that even higher amounts could increase the benefits. (Inositol is considered to be perfectly safe, with no toxic dosage.)

Taking this amount of inositol in capsule form is a tall order especially if you have difficulty in swallowing pills. (There is also the question of bioavailability.) Inositol is also available in a powdered form that can be stirred into water or juice, although you may have trouble controlling the exact amount unless you have a pharmaceutical scale.

A third option is a new effervescent formulation of powdered inositol, which is packaged in premeasured 4-gram packets. Effervescent delivery systems for vitamins and other nutrients are very popular in Europe and Asia. This method eliminates the question of whether capsules are fully dissolving in your stomach and is believed to produce a more sustained release of nutrients into the blood stream.

Powdered and capsule forms of inositol are readily available from health-food stores or through mail-order sources. The effervescent formulation is not yet available through retail outlets, but can be ordered from the source listed on page 149.

Actions:
- Regulates serotonin levels in the brain
- Plays important role in nerve cell communication

Benefits:
- Appears to help conditions that don't respond to SSRIs
- No unpleasant side effects including nausea, headaches, insomnia, and a reduced sex drive
- Improves language and orientation in Alzheimer's patients
- Manages OCD symptoms
- Decrease frequency and severity of panic attacks
- Relieves depression

21

Kava Kava:
The Feel-Good Herb of the South Pacific

Though kava kava has been around for thousands of years and is widely used as a pharmaceutical in Europe, few in America are keyed in to what this herb can do.

Kava kava (Piper methysticum) is a member of the pepper family. This lush, green plant with heart-shaped leaves grows as high as 8 feet tall before being harvested by the South Pacific islanders.

Islanders drink the pungent juice of the root instead of alcohol at bars. They take kava kava breaks instead of coffee breaks. They drink kava kava juice to celebrate wedding ceremonies. Feuding families drink it to remain calm, helping to resolve their problems. The elderly drink the juice to enhance mental clarity and to relax their muscles. And legend has it that a half coconut shell full of strong kava kava may put you into a deep, dreamless sleep for two hours.

If you have trouble falling asleep, if you wake up in the middle of the night and can't get back to sleep, or if you sleep fitfully all night and rise in the morning feeling exhausted...kava kava may be the answer to your prayers.

A potent treatment for serious and disruptive anxiety-related disorders

Make no mistake, this natural intoxicant is also a serious—but safe—herbal medicine. It is used to treat...

- depression
- anxiety and panic attacks
- insomnia
- mood swings

As a natural relaxant that reduces stress, kava kava is also helpful for high blood pressure. And, because it has been shown to have analgesic properties, it may help to relieve any painful condition—headaches, toothaches, and general muscle pain.

A proven folk medicine—backed up by 150 years of research

Proof of kava kava's effectiveness and safety is supported by hundreds (if not thousands) of years of use by the island communities of the South Pacific—from Hawaii to New Zealand. In addition, Western scientific studies on kava kava date as far back as the mid 1800s, when European scientists first began to identify, isolate, and test what they discovered to be the active ingredients: kavalactones.

Although the kava kava plant contains at least 15 different kavalactones, 150 years of research has shown that only six are biochemically active: yangonin, methysticin, kavain, dihydromethysticin (DHM), dihydrokavakavain, and demethosy-yangonin.

It is through these lipidlike substances that kava kava works its gentle magic.

A potent alternative to prescription sleep aids and antidepressants

As is evident from the popularity of Prozac (the first-ever $2 billion-dollar antidepressant) and the growing class of antianxiety drugs known as benzodiazepines (such as Valium, Halcion, Xanax, and Serax), Americans are in need of a safe, natural mood-relaxing substance.

As many as 22.2 percent of women and 16.9 percent of men in the United States suffer from anxiety disorders, according to the National Foundation for Brain Research.

During any six-month period, 9 million Americans suffer from a depressive illness, says the National Institutes of Mental Health.

It is estimated that 60 percent of American adults experience some degree of sleeplessness as a result of either depression or anxiety. Benzodiazepines, the most commonly prescribed antianxiety drugs, can cause headaches, drowsiness, dizziness, and vertigo and are physically habit-forming. In addition, their effects often diminish over time, making it necessary to increase the dosage.

Kava kava, on the other hand, is nonaddictive and nontoxic when taken at the recommended dosage. Research has proven that kavakava works and that it's safe

A number of studies have shown that kavakava relaxes the limbic system, the emotional center of the brain. Like the benzodiazepines, kavalactones act on the small, chickpea-sized organ called the amygdala, which regulates feelings of fear and anxiety and processes memories en route to the cerebral cortex.

Researchers have yet to explain, however, how kava kava produces its relaxing and uplifting response without the side effects and hazards of prescription antianxiety drugs. But they do know this:

- Kava kava is as strong as prescription antianxiety drugs, but with NO side effects. In 1990, a team of German researchers conducted a four-week study that compared the effects of kava kava and oxazapam (a popular benzodiazepine) on 38 patients suffering from anxiety. The kava kava extract reduced symptoms of anxiety as effectively as oxazapam—but with no side effects.

- Kava kava does not inhibit mental function. In 1993, researchers made use of standardized tests for mental function and reaction time to compare kava kava with benzodiazepine. The study demonstrated that while the benzodiazepine decreased both the quality and the speed of responses to test questions, the kava kava reduced anxiety without interfering with mental clarity. In fact, those who took the kava kava had slightly improved reaction time and recognition.

- Kava kava outperforms placebos. In a 1991 study of 58 patients with anxiety, researchers gave half the patients 100 milligrams of a 70 percent kavalactone extract three times a day for four weeks. The other half (the control group) received placebos. Those who took the kava kava extract enjoyed significant relief from their symptoms in just one week. (No side effects were reported.)

- Kava kava is an effective painkiller. While it was already well-known that chewing fresh kava kava produced local anesthesia in the chewer's mouth, a team of scientists from the Freiburg University Institute of Pharmacology in Germany, led by J. Meyer, established that one kavalactone in particular, kavain, functions as a superficial anesthetic, as effective as cocaine but completely nontoxic to the tissues.

Kava kava has also proven to help reduce symptoms of depression and anxiety in menopausal women.

Take a lesson—and a cure—from the ancient wisdom of the South Pacific

You can mix kava kava tinctures with herbal tea, take the extract as a capsule or tablet, or take the liquid form under your tongue. (The liquid form works faster, but it may not last as long.) To make sure you're getting an effective dose and product, look for a standardized kava kava extract containing at least 25 to 30 percent kavalactones.

It's not dangerous to take an unstandardized supplement, but you won't be able to determine the exact potency and may have to take more of the product to get the desired results.

Though kava kava is readily available in health-food stores, biochemist Herman Lam recently introduced a high-potency extract to the American Academy of Environmental Medicine:

I studied a number of different kava kava products, but none was as potent as I'd read it should be. When I finally found a product that worked—the Guaranteed Potency Extract—I introduced it at a medical meeting of the American Academy of Environmental Medicine in Boston. We didn't have the capsule form yet, so I offered samples of the liquid variety. Five or six doctors expressed interest in the product, but they were also concerned—they didn't want to fall asleep. I promised it wouldn't put them to sleep, filled their glasses...and a few minutes later, one doctor sang out that her headache was gone. Another said that his back pain disappeared. It went on and on...the crowd got larger and larger...

Recommended amount of kava kava

Though native islanders drink it by the coconut shell, Western science has provided a dosage range for the uninitiated—between 70 and 250 milligrams of kavalactones. Try 70 milligrams for a mild relaxing effect; increase the dosage to 150-250 as a sleep aid.

In terms of standardized supplements, if the preparation you buy contains, for example, 150 mg of standardized kava kava root extract, at 30 percent kavalactones, you're getting 50 mg of kavalactones.

A word of caution: Overindulgence in kava kava (310 to 440 grams per week) may lead to liver damage, dry scaly skin, and alterations in red and white blood cells and platelets. (A 1988 study in Australia showed that heavy kava kava drinkers suffered from malnutrition because the kava kava consumption replaced much of the subjects' food intake.)

For information on the availability of kava kava, see the "Guide to Sources and Availability" on page 149.

Actions:
- Relaxes the limbic system, the emotional center of the brain
- Regulate feeling of fear and anxiety
- Acts as a natural analgesic

Benefits:
- Reduces stress
- Calms anxiety and panic attacks
- Prevents insomnia
- Relieves pain
- Does not inhibit mental function

SECTION VI
Super Sex for as Long as You Want

Although perhaps rarely discussed, even between the closest of couples, and almost never by the medical establishment, loss of libido is one of the most disturbing effects of aging. Even the American Medical Association's *Encyclopedia of Medicine* defines libido (sex drive) as something that can be expected to fade with age. But satisfactory and exciting sexual vigor can be maintained into old age, and this section highlights three breakthrough products that can help without the risks and unknowns of Viagra.

22

V-Power: Promote Your Sexual Health

For many men, as they age, maintaining prime sexual function is a primary concern. To do this, you first need a healthy heart and cardiovascular condition. In the heart-health section of this book, you can read about how nutritional supplements can help keep your arteries youthful and flexible. But you also need to have powerful, local circulation...plenty of blood flowing strongly into your penis. And there are ways to increase both general and local circulation—without risking your life with drugs like Viagra.

There are dozens of herbs reputed to be sexual stimulants, but two in particular have been proven in modern, scientific trials to increase blood flow to the penis.

Coleus forskohlii is an herb from India that dilates the arteries going to your penis, increasing blood supply to the region. It also blocks a certain enzyme that is known to suppress your ability to form an erection. This effective and targeted approach to impotence has been the model for pharmaceutical impotence drugs. But the all-natural original has one important advantage: It is perfectly safe, and it even promotes healthy blood-pressure levels.

Muira Puama (also known as Amazon Potency Wood) is another natural substance proven to enhance sexual function. A study by French researchers found that more than 50% of men suffering from erectile dysfunction reported improvement when using it.

Poor circulation is at the root of many sexual problems, and it is relatively easy to address by using natural substances like Forskohlin, and Muira Puama. But circulation is only the beginning of the story. Often, when circulatory problems that cause impotence are corrected, another underlying problem surfaces: a diminished sex drive, or lack of desire for sex. And that's something you won't hear about from the folks promoting Viagra, because Viagra can't do a thing to enhance a reduced libido.

Testosterone—fueling the fire

A lagging libido, or a reduced desire for sex, is the second most common form of sexual dysfunction and is usually the result of low

> ### Viagra: Does it work? Is it safe?
>
> Viagra helps impotent men achieve erections by causing tiny blood vessels in the penis to relax, allowing blood to flow in and cause an erection. It does work—about half the time. But it's not safe. According to reports filed with the Food and Drug Administration, the drug has been linked to heart attacks and can be fatal when combined with common heart medication like nitrates (used for angina pain). If you have any kind of cardiac disorder or other risk factor or are taking cardiac medications, you should not be taking Viagra.
>
> Viagra can also damage your vision, reducing your retinal function by up to 50% for several hours after use...and possibly permanently. It can cause extreme light sensitivity and cause a pronounced blue tint in your field of vision. The American Academy of Ophthalmology has issued warnings about the serious risks of Viagra.
>
> More importantly, in order for Viagra to work for you, you must suffer from erectile dysfunction due only to insufficient blood flow to the penis. If you wake up in the morning with an erection but rarely have the energy or drive for sex, then Viagra is almost sure to disappoint.
>
> And if you are simply looking for a sex aid to enhance your pleasure, you're looking in the wrong place. If you can already achieve and maintain an erection, Viagra is not going to enhance your performance or staying power.
>
> Viagra does one thing and one thing only—it causes blood to flow to, and stay, in the penis. It does NOT:
>
> - Enhance your desire
> - Heighten your enjoyment
> - Give you the mental energy and alertness to perform optimally
> - Supply the physical vigor and stamina that fuels good sex

testosterone levels. According to some estimates, as many as 20 percent of men over 50 have testosterone levels below the normal range.

As we age, testosterone levels tend to decrease, but their decline is hastened in our modern society by the high amounts of estrogenlike chemicals in our environment. Pesticides, plastics, and other industrial chemicals pose a hidden threat to the modern male by throwing the body's hormones—especially sex hormones—out of balance.

In recent years, testosterone-replacement therapy has become

(Continued on page 118)

Keeping the prostate healthy

One of the more common health complaints for middle-aged and older men is a prostate problem. Sooner or later, it seems that prostate difficulties inevitably interfere with men's quality of life. At least six out of 10 men over the age of 50 have "significant" enlargement of the prostate, the doghnut-shaped gland that surrounds the urethra at the base of the penis.

The condition comes about when cells in the prostate begin to multiply too quickly, causing the prostate to swell, sometimes pressing on or pinching off the urethra. Benign prostatic hyperplasia, or BPH can cause pain and tenderness, painful or frequent urination, and can increase your risk of a prostatic disease like prostatitis (infection of the prostate gland) or even prostate cancer. And it can throw a wet blanket over even the healthiest sex life.

The prevention of prostatic disease is of primary importance. At all costs, you want to avoid prostate surgery, which can leave you permanently impotent and incontinent. But there is no reason to suffer a diminished quality of life or even occasional discomfort.

Prostate health can be easily enhanced and protected with simple nutritional measures. You may be familiar with saw palmetto, an herb that is commonly used to reduce swelling and inflammation of the prostate gland.

Saw palmetto works by blocking the action of an enzyme called 5-alpha-reductase. This leads to a reduction in the levels of dihydrotestosterone (DHT), a hormone that promotes growth of prostate tissue. It works by the same mechanism as synthetic pharmaceutical drugs for BPH—only better and with fewer side effects.

Other tried and true herbs for prostate health include:

Pygeum africanum is a powerful, natural anti-inflammatory that helps to reduce swelling of the prostate gland. Like saw palmetto, Pygeum has a well-established track record against BPH. In fact, French doctors regularly prescribe it for their patients suffering from BPH instead of pharmaceutical drugs.

Stinging nettle possesses strong anti-inflammatory properties and also helps regulate sex-hormone levels in the prostate. Studies show that it can reduce the size of a swollen prostate by over 50 percent.

Recent research has led to new breakthroughs in the natural approach to prostate health. Scientists have uncovered two new

(continued on next page)

> *(continued from previous page)*
>
> power nutrients that substantially reduce the risk of malignant growth in the prostate.
>
> A recent study at the Harvard Medical School found that men with increased consumption of tomatoes and tomato products had a significantly lower risk of prostate cancer. Subsequent research isolated an antioxidant called lycopene as the active plant chemical responsible for this protective effect.
>
> The other breakthrough finally solved the mystery of why prostate difficulties are almost unheard of in Japan. Those who consume soy on a daily basis cut their risk of prostate cancer by almost 70 percent over those who eat it only once a week or less. (This is not the first time that soy has been revealed as a cancer prventive food: Other research has demonstrated lower rates of colorectal, breast, lung, and gastric cancer among soy eaters.)
>
> Scientists have established that naturally occurring chemicals called isoflavones are responsible for soy's powerful cancer protective effects. The most well-researched of the soy isoflavones is called genistein: It's been shown to selectively kill cancer cells and prevent the formation of blood vessels that support tumor growth. Soy also has weak hormonal effects and helps to balance hormonal imbalances.
>
> There are dozens of prostate formulas available in health-food stores—most of them feature saw palmetto and Pygeum. We have found a formulation called Prostate Health Complex that includes those two ingredients as well as lycopene and soy isoflavone concentrate. See the "Guide to Sources and Availability" on page 152 for the source of Prostate Health Complex.

popular, and testosterone "precursors" like androstenedione have become widely available over-the-counter. But these solutions—especially when attempted without a doctor's supervision—are not without risk. Although they may temporarily increase your sex drive, they may also inadvertently feed prostate-cancer growth or cause other health problems. They also do not tend to result in permanent improvement in sexual function.

Instead, we turn again to the wisdom of traditional Asian and Indian medicine. It is no coincidence that in these cultures men regularly marry and father children well into their 70s and 80s. For centuries, these cultures have used herbs to safely and naturally balance sex hormones and increase testosterone production, without any of the hazards of hormone therapy.

Three scientifically proven power herbs give the most significant boost to a sagging sex drive:

Tribulus terrestis is traditionally used in Ayurvedic (Indian) medicine as a male tonic—to improve the health of the prostate, penis, and urinary tract. More recent studies show that it leads to a significant increase (up to 30%) in testosterone levels in as little as five days. Men report that Tribulus not only steps up sex drive but also increases stamina and endurance; it's helpful in the bedroom as well as the in the gym or on the job.

Epimedium grandiflorum is used in Chinese medicine to combat impotence and infertility. Clinical research has shown that it acts directly on the testes and prostate gland, increasing sperm production, and stimulates the sensory nerves that can trigger sexual desire.

Ginseng has long been revered for its potency and libido-enhancing powers. Panax ginseng has been found to increase sperm production and raise testosterone levels and is considered one of the most potent herbal libido enhancers.

These herbs, along with the circulation-enhancing herbs discussed earlier are best used together for the most reliable results. When using herbs in combination, however, it is important to adjust the amounts accordingly. Because each enhances the action of the others, you can get the maximum benefit from smaller amounts than you might use if you were taking them individually.

HSI researchers have uncovered a libido and potency formula called V-Power that includes all five of these powerful herbs—along with several other supporting nutrients—in the amounts found to be most effective in enhancing circulation, performance, and desire. V-Power is available from the source listed on page 152.

Actions:

- Increases blood flow to the penis
- Balances sex hormones and increases testosterone production

Benefit:

- Safe, natural sexual stimulant

23

Wild Yam Cream for Men and Women: Restore Optimum Hormone Levels

In the past 50 years, the world has been swamped with dangerous chemicals that we now know have serious health consequences for all of us. Many of these substances are "endocrine disrupters"—they disrupt the body's natural hormone balance by imitating the action of the natural hormone estrogen.

You can't avoid this chemical poisoning—the chemicals are simply too widespread. Some are commonly used in pesticides, fungicides, and insecticides; others show up in industrial chemicals, detergents, and food dyes. For example, red dye No. 3, added to hot dogs and other popular processed foods, emits an estrogen mimic.

Synthetic hormones are also created as byproducts in the manufacture of such everyday items as paper and plastics—the very plastics in which you may store your vitamins and wrap your foods; the plastics you sit on, cook with, eat with, and sleep on! The plastic coating in a single can of peas contains a powerful estrogen mimic, the action of which is 300 million times higher than the natural action of estradiol (the most potent form of estrogen).

Your body, mistaking the synthetic estrogens all around you for the real thing, accepts and processes them, day in and day out, until your hormone balance is thrown completely out of whack and your body is dangerously overloaded with unnatural sex hormones.

Attention, men: Estrogen isn't just a female hormone. Men produce it too, and, believe it or not, too much estrogen, whether you manufacture it or get it from the environment, increases your risk of prostate enlargement—just as too much testosterone has been implicated as one of the causes of prostate cancer.

Environmental estrogen may be the cause of many modern ills

Dozens of studies in the past few years have led researchers to the same conclusion: These chemicals lower sperm counts and contribute to the sharp increases in testicular and prostate cancer, as well as breast cancer and endometriosis. Rates of testicular cancer have doubled, tripled, and even quadrupled in some parts of the world in the last half of this century. Breast-cancer rates have increased by over 30 percent and prostate-cancer rates by 60 percent. Once a rare disease, endometriosis (a painful inflammation of the uterus that can cause sterility) now afflicts millions of women.

Incidence of abnormal pregnancy is on the rise. Average sperm counts worldwide have decreased by 50 percent in the past 50 years. Many researchers believe that the widespread exposure to estrogen disrupters in the fetal stage 50 years ago contributed to our currently high rates of infertility and sex-organ cancers. HSI panel members believe that lifetime exposure to estrogen mimics is a major cause of this epidemic of hormone-related diseases and disorders. You can't avoid these chemicals, but you can defend your body against their damaging effects.

You can rebalance your hormone ratios

The phenomenal success of natural progesterone therapy has been documented and validated over and over again. Don't confuse this with prescribed synthetic progestins. We are referring to cream-based products that contain a blend of wild Mexican yam (which exhibits progesterone-type activity), a small amount of natural progesterone, and synergistic herbs. This combination appears to provide optimal benefit without the hazards associated with other popular hormone therapies.

Progesterone also favors the development of T cells in both men and women, thereby boosting immunity. It increases dopamine release, supplying a good precursor for adrenal hormones—again, for both sexes. Progesterone is a primary hormone responsible for the manufacture of other hormones, including cortisone. Cortisone works to reduce inflammation and suppress unwanted immune-system responses. This means that it can help with arthritis pain. It also has the overall effect of helping your body deal with stressful psychological situations.

For women: an alternative to hormone-replacement therapy

The dangers of the conventional practice of prescribing synthetic hormone-replacement therapy for women are far more serious than generally recognized. Furthermore, the effectiveness of such therapy for reducing heart disease and osteoporosis has been seriously questioned.

A natural formula containing progesterone and herbs has the potential to relieve PMS and menopausal symptoms, including irritability, hot flashes, water retention, vaginal dryness, fatigue, and mood swings and

> ### Progesterone cream can relieve arthritis pain
>
> When you supply your body with adequate amounts of progesterone, you may be able to restore cortisone levels to normal and to reduce—even eliminate—arthritic inflammation. Helpful for both rheumatoid arthritis and osteoarthritis, the most effective progesterone products contain a small amount of this hormone plus a few herbs with progesterone-type activity, including the now famous Mexican wild yam.
>
> #### Protects against osteoporosis in both men and women
>
> In both men and women, progesterone protects against osteoporosis by working directly on cells called osteoblasts, which actually build new bone.
>
> Keep in mind that estrogen therapy does not reverse osteoporosis. It merely reduces the rate of bone loss by affecting the activity of osteoclasts, the cells that cause calcium to leach out of your bones and reenter your blood plasma. And if the estrogen is synthetic, the reduction in bone loss is only temporary.
>
> Again and again, it's been demonstrated that after six months to a year of natural progesterone use, bone density can be increased even in women who are 70 and over.

help to protect against breast cancer, fibrocysts, and endometriosis. It also supports thyroid hormone actions, normalizes zinc and copper levels, normalizes blood clotting and blood-sugar levels, helps use fat for energy, and, according to endless anecdotal reports, may even restore lost libido.

We've found a good formula for women that contains chamomile, burdock root, black cohosh, and Siberian ginseng—in addition to wild yam extract, a small amount of natural progesterone, and special oils to facilitate absorption and even moisturize the skin. The application of this cream, when properly formulated, has been shown to play an important role in hormonal balance.

What's in wild yam cream for women?

- Black cohosh—improves mood, relieves painful migraine headaches, and reduces hot flashes and vaginal dryness
- Burdock root—Detoxifies your body and supports your immune system, so your hormones work at capacity and the hormonal

"roller coaster ride" is diminished
- Siberian ginseng—Increases energy, enhances sexual desire and helps you handle stress
- Chamomile—Calms you down and helps maintain normal menstrual flow, reducing spotting and erratic periods

Health Sciences Institute researchers have found that, in most cases, the need for hormones suggests a hormone imbalance, which does not occur in isolation. In other words, a hormone imbalance suggests a decline in other systems as well. That's why stabilizing agents like herbs are recommended to supplement hormone therapy.

A progesterone preparation designed specifically for men

HSI panelist Dr. Howard Bezoza has tried administering testosterone therapy to men and has concluded that "believe it or not, testosterone therapy doesn't always raise hormonal levels. I've tried it with many men—in oral capsules, cream, and patches. And it creates a symphony of problems. Where most doctors go wrong is in measuring the single androgen (testosterone) and not measuring the whole picture. They miss the boat.

There are too many other factors. Often these men have lower levels of other hormones as well, hormones like pregnenolone, DHEA, and estrogens that increase the risk of prostate problems."

A special men's wild yam cream formula containing progesterone and synergistic herbs has the potential to improve sperm quality and quantity and boost potency. It may shrink enlarged prostates and may protect against prostate and testicular cancer as well.

What's in wild yam cream for men?
- Herbs that work synergistically with progesterone: Siberian ginseng—enhances a feeling of general well being and stimulates and keeps the testes and the prostate healthy
- Saw palmetto—boosts the function of the testes and keep free testosterone from breaking down into DHT, a substance known to encourage prostate enlargement
- Wild oat straw (avina sativa)—increases libido
- Damiana—a potent general tonic, damiana is a safe and popular aphrodisiac
- Ginkgo biloba—stimulates and enhances blood circulation and

boosts mental performance. Can also help reverse impotency caused by poor circulation in the lower pelvis
- Gotu kola—enhances mental function, improves mood, and helps to maintain a positive, focused arousal

A little progesterone goes a long way!

In the case of hormones, more is not always better. In fact, you need only a small amount of progesterone to get the desired results. If you're using one of the high-dose preparations (some have as much as 900 or more milligrams of progesterone in a 2-ounce jar), it is advisable to be under a doctor's care. You need to be monitored periodically to be sure that you are not getting too much of a good thing! Recent laboratory results indicate that high doses of progesterone can lead to an accumulation of hormones in your tissues.

The lower-dose preparations—usually 10 milligrams per 2-ounce jar—are safer, and they are just as effective for most men and women when prepared with the synergistic herbs described above. Recommended usage of the low-dose cream is one-eighth to one-half teaspoon a day. A 2-ounce jar should last one to two months. For purchasing information, see page 150 for the "Guide to Sources and Availability."

Actions:
- Provides building blocks for other hormones
- Helps maintain optimum hormone balance in reproductive and sex-related organs
- May favor the development of T cells in both men and women

Benefits:
- Increases energy
- Normalizes libido
- Helps the body use fat for energy
- Alleviates inflammation and pain
- Protects against osteoporosis by facilitating new bone growth
- Reduces the risks associated with an estrogen overload
- Relieves depression
- Stabilizes mood
- Boosts immunity

24

RED DEER ANTLER VELVET: ANIMALLIKE RESULTS

An ancient scroll recommends deer antler for 52 different diseases. Today, it has been scientifically proven to strengthen muscle contractions, improve nerve impulses, regulate blood pressure, and treat arthritis.

Deer antler velvet sounds like the kind of ingredient that should go into the cauldron right after "eye of newt" and just before "toe of frog." At first impression, the uninformed might be tempted to put the users of antler products on the "far out" nutritional fringe. And yet this substance has a credible history of effective use in Chinese herbal medicine that goes back at least two millennia, and it continues to be widely used in China, Korea, Japan, and Russia.

What is antler velvet?

We think of the antler as an inert growth of material with no biological activity. This is more or less true, but the velvet is an entirely different kind of tissue than the actual antler material itself.

Male deer grow a new set of antlers every year. Unlike most mammalian tissue, which contains an internal circulatory system to provide blood and nutrients, the blood flow to new antlers is on the outside of the antlers. The velvet is a fuzzy membrane that contains and distributes this external supply of blood and nutrients to support the new antler's growth. And this growth rate is extremely rapid: on a large male, a 20-pound set of antlers can grow in three to four months. The velvet falls off as mating season approaches, and the fully mineralized antlers become the inert structures we perceive them to be.

So the antler velvet, in sharp contrast to the antlers themselves, is a tissue of extremely high and specialized bioactivity. It is rich with precursors for growth hormone, leutinizing hormone (the hormone stimulating testosterone synthesis), and prostaglandins. It contains elements that could be effective against cancer and arthritis, similar to those found in shark cartilage.

How does it work?

It's not surprising that several modes of action are at work with such a complicated substance. Some of the therapeutic properties of red deer antler velvet appear to be similar to those of cartilage. Of particular interest, however, is the relatively high level of insulinlike growth factor found in deer antler.

Growth hormones have an anabolic effect. That is, they cause tissue to grow and cause stored energy (fat) to be consumed. This is in contrast to hormones that are catabolic, causing tissue to break down and release energy—an endocrinological dichotomy that is reminiscent of the yang and yin of Chinese medicine.

Insulin, the hormone released by the pancreas to help metabolize sugar, is also anabolic. Some of the effects of growth hormone are similar to those of insulin, but others are in conflict. Growth hormone can impair glucose uptake in cells by suppressing the action of insulin receptors, while at the same time causing fatty acids to be released from fatty tissue.

A receptor is a special part of a cell, usually a protein in the cell membrane. It is "tuned in" to respond to the presence of a particular hormone and then initiate a process within the cell-like a radio receiver that only gets one station. In the case of insulinlike growth hormone, the hormone "looks" enough like insulin to jam the receiver, preventing regular "insulin signals" from getting through.

The net effect of the two actions(the suppression of insulin reception and the release of stored fat) is to encourage cells to consume fat rather than sugar or other carbohydrates, with obvious benefits for both bodybuilders and weight watchers.

Growth hormone also has an important role in immunity. The real nuts and bolts of immunity take place at the cell-membrane level, where specialized proteins "float" in the thin fatty membrane, controlling what goes in and what goes out. For at least part of the day, it's critical to maintain a protein-building (anabolic) environment: If you can build protein, you can strengthen your immune system; if you are consuming protein to maintain blood sugar or other crucial physiological functions, immunity gradually degrades. So the daily production of growth hormone is enormously important, especially as we age.

Unfortunately, growth-hormone production falls off very quickly as we leave our teen years. Between the ages of 20 and 23, daytime growth-hormone levels begin to drop. And by the time we reach age 30, even the growth-hormone release in response to vigorous exercise is greatly reduced.

Much of the action of growth hormone is carried out through

secondary hormones called somatomedins. These hormones are manufactured in the liver in response to growth hormone, and the two main somatomedins promote bone growth, collagen synthesis, and the stimulation of tissue growth.

In an older individual with very low growth-hormone production, a natural dietary source of these hormones has been shown to produce the same anabolic effects found in a much younger individual. This is probably the best way to account for the reported rejuvenating properties of deer antler velvet. In addition to the beneficial growth hormones, the following substances are also found in red deer antler velvet:

- prostaglandins, which help control a wide range of physiological functions, including reduction of inflammation—especially important to athletes and arthritis sufferers
- velvatins, which include a nucleoside demonstrated to have value in cancer therapy and AIDS treatment. Nucleosides are the building blocks of DNA and RNA, the masters of cellular function
- pantocrine, shown in a 1974 Russian study by Dr. Arcady Koltun to increase athletic performance
- N-acetyl-glucosamine sulfate, for wound healing
- chondroitin sulfate, which, along with glucosamine, is an effective agent against arthritis. (Chondroitin sulfate in particular has been claimed to reverse atherosclerosis and dramatically improve circulation)

Traditional Chinese medicine calls for its use to treat impotence and

---

What is red deer antler used for?

In Korea and Japan, red deer antler velvet is commonly used to:
- increase blood production in the treatment of anemia
- modulate the immune system
- treat infertility in women
- treat impotence in men
- improve blood circulation in patients with heart disease
- improve muscle tone and glandular functions
- increase lung efficiency
- increase muscular strength and nerve function

infertility, frequent urination, cold extremities, lower back and knee pain, loss of hearing, tinnitus (ringing in the ears), and dizziness.

Future uses are likely to include treatment of a wide range of degenerative diseases, especially arthritis. It continues to show great promise as a natural source of growth-hormone precursors, useful for achieving both athletic and weight-reduction goals.

Data and research, published and otherwise

Despite its long history of medicinal use, authoritative studies on the use of this product are scarce. But there are a few exceptions. Research from 1989 (by Dr. Ivan Kinia) shows that constituents of deer antler velvet are anti-inflammatory.

A Russian study (Dr. Taneyvia, 1964) claims to demonstrate that young men score better on intelligence tests after using velvet deer antler.

In Japan, a 1988 report by Dr. Wang showed that red deer antler increases the number of blood components related to the immune system.

In New Zealand, studies at the Invermay Research Center indicate that antler extracts improve cell growth and have antitumor and antiviral properties.

And in China, researchers at the Chinese Academy of Medical Sciences in Beijing found that nutrients in deer antler increased the number of cell replications by a factor of three, from about 60 to 180.

Is it only for males?

Both male and female hormones are found in deer antler velvet. It is equally beneficial for both sexes.

Animal friendliness

In modern times, many antler products are regarded as "elite" natural remedies (partly due to their scarcity and expense but also because of the uncomfortable opposition between the concern for endangered species and the interest in natural healing).

In the case of deer antler velvet, modern harvesting methods do not affect wild populations and do not destroy any animals. In fact, no pain or stress to the deer is evident even when the antler itself is removed, suggesting that this could be a useful "animal-friendly" alternative for obtaining nutritional substances that are difficult to get from other sources. (Other parts of the antler are also used as nutritional supplements. The antler, however, is the only appendage that can be regenerated by advanced mammals.)

See the "Guide to Sources and Availability" on page 152 for the source of red deer antler velvet.

Actions:
- Impairs glucose uptake in cells by suppressing the action of insulin receptors
- Causes fatty acids to be released from fatty tissues
- Helps maintain a protein-building (anabolic) environment
- Promotes the manufacture of somatomedins (secondary growth hormones) in the liver

Benefits:
- Encourages cells to consume fat rather than sugar or other carbohydrates
- Helps strengthen the immune system
- Stimulates bone growth, collagen synthesis, and tissue growth

SECTION VII
Powerful Pain-Relief Solutions

Like most people living with pain caused by arthritis, injury, migraines or surgery, you have probably tried everything to bring some relief, reluctant to become dependent on painkillers or barbiturates to get through the day. The products in this section are natural, nontoxic, nonaddictive solutions discovered by the Health Sciences Institute. See also organic germanium on page 63 for an additional breakthrough product for pain.

25

XP-100™:
A GENTLE ALTERNATIVE TO IBUPROFEN

If you go to your doctor with pain, he will probably recommend either a pain reliever like aspirin or Tylenol or a nonsteroidal anti-inflammatory drug (NSAID) like ibuprofen. These may temporarily mask the pain, but they won't solve the problem, and they can make you very sick. These—and stronger prescription drugs like steroids—carry serious and immediate long-term risks to your health. In fact, NSAIDs account for an estimated 7,600 deaths and 76,000 hospitalizations each year.[1] And with no better treatments being offered, it's no wonder that arthritis is considered an incurable condition.

The problems with using NSAIDs in the treatment of arthritis are numerous:

- NSAIDs work by blocking production of prostaglandins, hormonelike substances in your body that can promote pain and inflammation. The problem is that they also block good prostaglandins, those that are responsible for some very important bodily functions, including blood-pressure regulation, gastric-acid secretion, and blood clotting.

- Side effects of NSAID use include hypertension, digestive difficulties, ulcers, stomach bleeding[2], kidney disease[3], and liver disease[4], among the most serious.

- The segment of the population at greatest risk for osteoarthritis, that is, the elderly, appears to be at greater risk than younger individuals for gastrointestinal symptoms, ulceration, hemorrhage, and death as a result of inhibition of the synthesis of protective prostaglandins.[5]

- By alleviating pain and inflammation, NSAIDs can disguise or "mask" your arthritis symptoms, so the disease continues

---

[1] *Annals of Internal Medicine*, vol. 127, p. 429, 1997.
[2] *New England Journal of Medicine*, vol. 331, no. 25, pp. 1675-1679, 1994
[3] *Annals of Internal Medicine*, vol. 109, pp. 359-363, 1988
[4] *Annals of Internal Medicine*, vol. 114, no. 4, pp. 257-263, 1991
[5] *Gastroenterology*, vol. 96, supp. 2, pp. 647-675, 1989

unchecked, even while you may be feeling better.[6]
- There is evidence that NSAIDs may inhibit the production of proteoglycans, the molecules that attract water to cartilage. In this way, NSAIDs may actually hasten the progression of arthritis.
- NSAIDs can interact with blood pressure-medicine, altering its effectiveness with potentially dangerous consequences to your health.

Despite the potential for dire consequences from NSAIDs and steroids, more doctors are prescribing them than ever before, especially in the treatment of rheumatoid arthritis. There's a reason for this: They are somewhat effective in alleviating debilitating pain and inflammation. But we have found safer alternatives to these dangerous drugs.

Powerful pain relief from an amino acid

XP-100™ contains as its active ingredient a naturally occurring amino acid that may help your body unlock its own healing and pain-relieving powers. The ingredient—called phenylalanine—may well provide you with the most complete pain relief you have ever experienced, without any adverse side effects.

Phenylalanine is readily available in foods and is essential for many bodily functions. It is also one of the few amino acids that can cross the blood-brain barrier and thus directly affect brain chemistry.

In arthritis, the DL form of phenylalanine provides pain relief naturally, through its function of increasing endorphins in the brain. DL-phenylalanine blocks the enkephalinase enzymes that break down the endorphins and enkephalins, natural pain relievers and mood elevators. (Many patients report an increased feeling of well-being in addition to their pain relief.)

XP-100™ is a natural pain reliever that you can use instead of NSAIDs for everything from arthritis pain to headaches. And the natural pain relief from XP-100™ lasts up to five full days. No major side effects have been noted, and it is safe to use in conjunction with your medications. In fact, you can safely use it in combination with other pain relievers to boost their effects. You may also use it to reduce your reliance on NSAIDs.

Impressive results are reported from a major clinical study at the

---

[6] *Journal of the American Geriatric Society*, vol. 17, pp. 710-717, 1969

University of Chicago Medical School. In this study, the main ingredient in XP-100™ was given to people suffering pain. And every single subject who was given this substance experienced good to excellent relief.

Consider the story of the 29-year-old man suffering from whiplash pain who had been treated for two years with aspirin and Valium—with unsatisfactory results. When he was given the special amino acid, he experienced complete relief from pain. Another success story is that of a 64-year-old woman suffering form osteoarthritis in her hands who had been treated with aspirin for five years with unsatisfactory results. When she was given this special amino acid, she not only experienced relief from pain but also noted a marked reduction in her joint stiffness.

If you suffer from most any type of pain, whether it is arthritis, migraine, PMS, muscle pain, or mouth pain, you may benefit from XP-100™. For sources of this all-natural pain-relieving substance, see page 152.

Actions:

- Helps the body unlock its own healing and pain-relieving powers
- Allows the body's own painkilling substances, which are 18 to 50 times stronger than morphine, to banish pain

Benefits:

- Not habit-forming
- Not harmful to the stomach
- Increases the effectiveness of other pain relievers such as aspirin and acupuncture
- Lasts much longer than aspirin or narcotics
* *Persons with PKU (Phenylkatonuria) and people with hypertension (high blood pressure) should consult a physician before taking any product that contains DL-phenylalanine*

26

The Farabloc Blanket: Banish Pain Without Drugs

Despite 26 years of testing, double-blind studies, joyful testimonials, and solid professional recommendations, this exciting product remains mysteriously unknown.

It even works on the most excruciating kinds of pain: crushed bones, spinal-column diseases, and even phantom limb pain—the very condition for which the fabric was invented.

The Farabloc blanket was developed in Bavaria by Frieder Kempe, a young inventor with a background in engineering and physics. Kempe was working to find a solution to the excruciating pain suffered by his father, an amputee.

Noting that his father's pain was worse on humid or rainy (low-pressure-system) days, Kempe theorized that positive atmospheric ions in the air were irritating the cut nerve endings in his father's stump. He reasoned that this external magnetic field was causing the nerve ends to send false signals to the brain—signals suggesting that the limb, along with the pain, was still there.

Over 50 different treatments had been tested on sufferers of phantom pain, and not one had worked well enough to be called a success: not surgery, drugs, ultrasound, hypnotherapy, psychotherapy, biofeedback—nothing.

After four years of research and development, Kempe tested the first prototype of the Farabloc blanket on his father. When the new invention eased his father's phantom pain, it was clear that Kempe's work had resulted in a revolution in pain relief.

After his initial success, Kempe set out to create a thinner, softer, more comfortable, and more durable fabric. He tested cotton and linen versions but found them both less durable than the fabric he'd originally chosen: nylon. The final version, available today, is made of microthin threads of stainless-steel wire woven with nylon. With proper care, this lightweight fabric, which looks and feels like linen, can last years.

Kempe named the fabric Farabloc after Michael Faraday, the 19th-century French scientist who discovered electromagnetic induction, which later led to the invention of electricity. (The farad, an electromagnetic unit, was named in his honor.)

After five more years of testing, Kempe applied for and received a U.S. patent for his fabric. He then offered samples to amputees in Bavaria. They claimed it gave them "remarkable relief" from their pain. Soon after, Kempe immigrated to Canada, where he established the Farabloc Development Corporation.

Today, thousands of amputees all over the world—including Kempe's father, still living in Bavaria—are enjoying relief. The fabric has since been scientifically proven effective.

Skeptical scientists "couldn't believe the data"

In 1989, the British Columbia Health Ministry funded a two-year double-blind crossover study (Conine, et al., 1993) at the University of British Columbia. The study was run by Tali Conine, DHSc, PT, a professor of physical therapy at the University of British Columbia's School of Rehabilitation Medicine, and Dr. Cecil Hershler, a medical doctor and electrical engineer specializing in physical and rehabilitation medicine. A significant 61 percent of the first group and 62 percent of the second group reported the greatest pain relief when using Farabloc.

"We were so skeptical," says Conine, "we couldn't believe the data. We were at a loss to explain it in terms that scientists today understand. It was the most difficult article I have written in my life."

In the past five years, many professional health organizations have begun regularly purchasing the Farabloc products—notably, the Insurance Corporation of British Columbia, the Ministry of Social Services, the Workers Compensation Board of Downsview, Ontario, and Veterans Affairs, Canada.

More independent studies are under way to determine how well Farabloc works for arthritis, delayed onset muscle soreness, and tendonitis, as well as sports-related injuries that cause swelling, especially in the knees and arms. Meanwhile, Dr. Gerhard Bach, a noted rheumatologist in the United States and Germany, has already established the use of Farabloc in other areas of pain relief.

The percentages listed below represent those who reported relief that was "good" or "very good":

- 81.3 percent: phantom pain
- 85.0 percent: arthroses (described as "painful disruptions of the

functions of joints")
- 86.7 percent: spinal-column syndrome (described as "static-degenerative changes to the spinal column ")
- 79.4 percent: other syndromes (shoulder-arm syndrome, soft-part rheumatism, posttraumatic complaints, and complaints related to neoplasia)
- 63.6 percent: chronic polyarthritis (an inflammatory-rheumatic disorder characterized by chronic pain, swelling, and a reduction in the function of several small or large joints and tendon sheaths)
- 58.3 percent: menstrual complaints

How it works

The truth is that Farabloc's painkilling action is still somewhat of a mystery. But there are a few working theories. As Kempe originally postulated, the blanket works to shield nerve endings from the aggravating effect of external electrical and magnetic fields.

Dr. Hershler, one of the doctors who led the first double-blind study on amputees, has also hypothesized that chronic pain is caused by alterations in blood flow deep within the muscles. He believes Farabloc may actually increase circulation, thereby causing pain relief.

But there is another theory—that a slightly more mysterious healing mechanism is at work.

The truth about pain

Flowing from every swollen, torn, or inflamed tissue in your body are energy currents that send your brain the message to "feel pain." The best way to stop pain is to make those energy currents pass right out of you before they make it to your brain.

Since the late 1700s, scientists have been aware that our bodies generate electricity. Today, thanks to modern technology, we can evaluate health states by measuring various electrical waves. In fact, measurements of electrical output can determine just how healthy you are.

For example, studying electrical impulses in your brain helps to discern whether or not your brain is functioning normally. The EEG (electroencephalograph) test is used to uncover this information. When brain tumors are present, variations from the normal brain waves announce their presence. The same is true of heart and muscle areas.

Scientists can even determine your sleep quality simply by measuring your "output" of delta waves, which are recorded in people who are enjoying a good, deep sleep.

Disperse pain currents with this "space age" pain reliever

As an electrically conductive fabric, Farabloc induces an electromagnetic field around the body (or around the limb for a local wrap). With the Farabloc fabric, the electrical "pain" energy generated within your body passes out of the body into the electromagnetic field of the blanket like an electrical ground or sink, thereby dissipating the energy that would otherwise travel up the sensory nerves as "pain."

What doesn't Farabloc work on?

Farabloc has not been shown to relieve pain caused by bruising, abrasion, or chronic fatigue.

What are the risks?

In a word, none. There is no risk to your health whatsoever, and there are no side effects.

Says Dr. Hershler, "I can be 100 percent sure that wrapping a Farabloc blanket around your limb does you no harm."

How to use it

To sustain pain relief, it is recommended that you begin using the fabric at the onset of pain. Wrap the garment, in two or three layers, around the painful area. Farabloc works best when placed directly on the skin and worn for a few hours from the time pain begins. In addition to wearing the Farabloc fabric as a blanket, you can sew it into socks, gloves, or sleeves, for example. You can even wash and air dry this thin, fine gray cloth (being careful not to wring it, to avoid damaging the fabric).

The fabric comes in four different sizes, which range from $70 for a handkerchief size to $260 for a small blanket. See page 148 for the "Guide to Sources and Availability."

Farabloc has been reported to relieve:

- joint pain
- rheumatic pain
- children's growing pains

- menstrual cramps
- sports injuries
- backache
- postsurgical pain
- pain caused by cancer migraines and other types of headache

Actions:
- Shields nerve endings format he aggravating effects of external electrical and magnetic fields
- Increases circulation, thereby causing pain relief
- Produces an electromagnetic field around the body to absorb the pain energy located within your body.

Benefits:
- Relieves joint pain
- Delays onset muscle soreness
- Relieves menstrual cramps
- Eases the pain of migraines and other types of headaches

27

MIGRAINE FORMULA:
RELIEF FROM MIGRAINES...NATURALLY

If you suffer from migraines, you know they're more than just a headache. It is estimated that 25% to 30% of women and 15% to 20% of men get migraine headaches, and if you're one of them, you're familiar with the "aura," the nausea, the throbbing and pounding pain, and the sensitivity to light and motion. You also know how hard they are to predict and to treat.

Commonly prescribed painkillers provide only temporary relief from pain, and some users experience even greater pain once the painkiller wears off. For some migraine sufferers, aspirin or acetaminophen may do the trick, but others may use a vasoconstrictor like ergotamine tartrate, which has the uncomfortable side effects of nausea and vomiting. Now you have more options: Recent European research shows that therapeutic doses of riboflavin significantly reduce the frequency of migraines by more than a third and cut down the frequency and length of pain when they do occur (*Neurology*, vol. 50, pp. 466-70, 1998). However, isolated high-potency riboflavin supplements are not widely available. The typical multivitamin includes 50 mg, far less than the 400 mg necessary to prevent migraine. HSI researchers have recently discovered a new all-natural migraine-relief formula that provides not only the optimal amount of riboflavin but also ingredients intended to specifically reduce migraines, including the following:

- **Feverfew**, an herb that contains anti-inflammatory parthenolides
- **Vitamin B_6**, which boosts serotonin levels (a deficiency of which is associated with increased incidence of migraines)
- **Magnesium citrate**, which calms the nervous system; a diet of processed foods and refined sugars contributes to deficiency in this important mineral
- **Willow bark**, a natural source of salicylate, an anti-inflammatory with analgesic properties
- **Ginger**, an herbal anti-inflammatory with natural calming effects

HSI panelist Dr. Ron Hoffman shared the experience of a patient who tried the new formula: "A 35-year-old female patient with a history of severe migraine headaches actually required a letter from me while traveling that enabled her to obtain intravenous Demerol-the only thing that would relieve her pain. I tried all other conventional migraine drugs for her. "Within two months of taking this formula, she no longer required Demerol. Within four months, her migraines were gone."

According to Dr. Hoffman, the formula is best used as a preventive regimen, one capsule twice daily. See your Source Directory on page 150 for availability.

Actions:
- Acts as an anti-inflammatory
- Acts as an analgesic
- Boosts serotonin levels

Benefit:
- Reduces the frequency of migraines

Guide to Sources and Availability

Due to their breakthrough, underground nature, many of the remedies presented in Underground Cures may not be readily available in health-food stores or other retail outlets. As a service to our readers, we have identified several high-quality, reliable sources for the products discussed in this book.

If you are interested in continuing to have access to the latest, most powerful discoveries and modern, underground treatments like the ones in this book, please turn to page 159 to find out how you can receive monthly Members Alerts from the Health Sciences Institute.

The foregoing chapters have not been evaluated by the U.S. Food and Drug Administration. This information is not intended to diagnose, treat, cure, or prevent any disease.

Anti-Homocysteine Products (Chapter 10)
Advanced Nutritional Products
1300 Piccard Drive, Suite 204
Rockville, MD 20850
Tel: (888) 436-7200 or (301) 987-9000
Fax: (301) 963-3886

Burgstiner's Thymic Formula (Chapter 13)
Preventive Therapeutics Inc.
P.O. Box 281
Snellville, GA 30078
Tel: (800) 556-5530 or (770) 409-0900
Fax: (770) 409-0110
www.thymic.com

Calcium elenolate (olive-leaf extract) (Chapter 1)
Advanced Nutritional Products
1300 Piccard Drive, Suite 204
Rockville, MD 20850
Tel: (888) 436-7200 or (301) 987-9000
Fax: (301) 963-3886

Smartbasics
1626 Union Street
San Francisco, CA 94123
Tel: (800) 878-6520 or (415) 749-3990
Fax: (415) 351-1348

DHA (Omega-3 fish oil) (Chapter 19)
Advanced Nutritional Products
1300 Piccard Drive, Suite 204
Rockville, MD 20850
Tel: (888) 436-7200 or (301) 987-9000
Fax: (301) 963-3886

Farabloc (Chapter 26)
Please note that the Food and Drug Administration has recently prohibited the Farabloc Corporation (based in Canada) from shipping the fabric to anyone living in the United States. Despite published double-blind studies; enthusiastic endorsements form physicians, insurance agencies, and consumer groups; and decades of side-effect-free use, the FDA has declared that there is insufficient evidence to "adequately demonstrate the safety and effectiveness of Farabloc technology". For more information, contact the Farabloc Development Corporation.

Farabloc Development Corporation
3030 Lincoln Av., #211
Coquitlam, BC, Canada V3B 6B4
Tel: (604) 941-8201
Fax: (604) 941-8065

Freeze-Frame (Chapter 11)
Planetary Publications
14700 W. Park Ave.
Boulder Creek, CA 95006
Tel: (831) 338-2161 or (800) 372-3100
Fax: (831) 338-9861

Glycalkaloid Cream (SkinAnswer)(Chapter 6)
CompassioNet
P.O. Box 710
Saddle River, NJ 07458
Tel: (800) 510-2010 or (201) 236-3900
Fax: (201) 236-0090

Infopeptides (Chapter 3)
Smartbasics
1626 Union St.
San Francisco, CA 94123
Tel: (800) 878-6520 or (415) 749-3990
Fax: (415) 351-1348

Inositol (Chapter 20)
Advanced Nutritional Products
1300 Piccard Drive, Suite 204
Rockville, MD 20850
Tel: (888) 436-7200 or (301) 987-9000
Fax: (301) 963-3886

Ipriflavone (OsteoSupport) (Chapter 15)
Advanced Nutritional Products
1300 Piccard Drive, Suite 204
Rockville, MD 20850
Tel: (888) 436-7200 or (301) 987-9000
Fax: (301) 963-3886

Kava Kava (Chapter 21)
Lifestar Millennium, Inc.
2175 E. Francisco Blvd., #A-2
San Rafael, CA 94901
Tel: (415) 457-1400 or (800) 858-7477
Fax: (415) 457-8887

Vitalmax Vitamins
710 E. Hillsboro Blvd., Suite 101
Deerfield Beach, FL 33441
Tel: (800) 349-6977 (for information)
(800) 815-5151 or (410) 810-7905 (for ordering)
Fax: (410) 810-0910 (for ordering)

Lactoferrin (Chapter 2)
Advanced Nutritional Products
1300 Piccard Drive, Suite 204
Rockville, MD 20850
Tel: (888) 436-7200 or (301) 987-9000
Fax: (301) 963-3886

Smartbasics
1626 Union St.
San Francisco, CA 94123
Tel: (800) 878-6520 or (415) 749-3990
Fax: (415) 351-1348

Larreastat (Chapter 17)
Herbal Technologies
2588 Progress Street, Suite 1
Vista, CA 92083
Tel: (800) 211-9619 or (760) 734-1899
Fax: (760) 734-1876

Migraine Support Formula (Chapter 27)
Advanced Nutritional Products
1300 Piccard Drive, Suite 204
Rockville, MD 20850
Tel: (888) 436-7200 or (301) 987-9000
Fax: (301) 963-3886

Modified Citrus Pectin (Chapter 5)
Advanced Nutritional Products
1300 Piccard Drive, Suite 204
Rockville, MD 20850
Tel: (888) 436-7200 or (301) 987-9000
Fax: (301) 963-3886

Natural Progesterone Cream (Chapter 23)
Advanced Nutritional Products
1300 Piccard Drive, Suite 204
Rockville, MD 20850
Tel: (888) 436-7200 or (301) 987-9000
Fax: (301) 963-3886

Natural EFX
100 N. Central Expressway, Suite 350
Richardson, TX 75080
Tel: (972) 644-7500
Fax: (972) 680-3322

Organic Germanium (Chapter 12)
Advanced Nutritional Products
1300 Piccard Drive, Suite 204
Rockville, MD 20850
Tel: (888) 436-7200 or (301) 987-9000
Fax: (301) 963-3886

Vitamin Connection
72 Main St.
Burlington, VT 05401
Tel: (802) 862-2590 or (800) 760-3020
Fax: (802) 862-2459
www.vitaminconnection.com

PC Spes (Chapter 7)
BotanicLab
2900-B Saturn St.
Brea, CA 92821
Tel: (800) 242-5555 or (714) 524-5533
Fax: (800) 752-3859 or (714) 524-5222

Phosphatidylserine (Brain Power Plus) (Chapter 18)
Advanced Nutritional Products
1300 Piccard Drive, Suite 204
Rockville, MD 20850
Tel: (888) 436-7200 or (301) 987-9000
Fax: (301) 963-3886

Phytochemicals (PhytoGuard) (Chapter 9)
Advanced Nutritional Products
1300 Piccard Drive, Suite 204
Rockville, MD 20850
Tel: (888) 436-7200 or (301) 987-9000
Fax: (301) 963-3886

Probiotics (Chapter 4)
Vitamin Research Products
3579 Highway 50 E.
Carson City, NV 89701
Tel: (800) 877-2447 or (702) 884-1300
Fax: (702) 884-1331

Prostate Health Complex (Chapter 22)
Advanced Nutritional Products
1300 Piccard Drive, Suite 204
Rockville, MD 20850
Tel: (888) 436-7200 or (301) 987-9000
Fax: (301) 963-3886

RA Spes (Chapter 16)
BotanicLab
2900-B Saturn St.
Brea, CA 92621
Tel: (800) 242-5555 or (714) 524-5533
Fax: (800) 752-3859 or (714) 524-5222

Red Deer Antler Velvet (Chapter 24)
Lifestar Millenium
2175 East Francisco Blvd. #A-2
San Rafael, CA 94901
Tel: (800) 858-7477 or (415) 457-1400
Fax: (415) 457-8887

Shark Cartilage (BeneJoint) (Chapter 14)
CompassioNet
P.O. Box 710
Saddle River, NJ 07458
Tel: (800) 510-2010 or (201) 236-3900
Fax: (201) 236-0090

Virility Formula (V-Power) (Chapter 22)
Advanced Nutritional Products
1300 Piccard Drive, Suite 204
Rockville, MD 20850
Tel: (888) 436-7200 or (301) 987-9000
Fax: (301) 963-3886

XP-100 (Phenylalanine) (Chapter 25)
Healthier YOU
PO Box 9515
Lake Worth, FL 33466-9515
Tel: (800) 350-7430 (mention code AGR01)
Fax: (561) 881-0227

Index

A

AIDS, 4, 14
Acetyl-L-carnitine, 101
Actinic keratoses, 31
Adaptogen, 64
Aflatoxins, 20
Ai-yeh, 87
Alzheimer's disease, 55, 97, 103, 105, 107
Analgesic, 112, 146
Anemia, 129
Animal safety, 130
Antiadhesive agent, 27
Anti-aging, 50
Antianxiety drugs, 110
Antibacterial agent, 21
Antibiotic agent, 3
Antibiotics, 3, 17
Anticarcinogenic, 50
Antidepressants, 110
Antibiotics, natural, 4
Antifungal agent, 3
Antihomocysteine products, 147
Anti-inflammatory, 12, 50, 78, 86, 89, 146
Antitumor agents, 39
Antiviral agent, 6
Anxiety, 109
Antioxidant, 10, 12, 50, 102
Arthritis, 14, 69, 75, 140
Arthritis Foundation, 75
Arthritis of the spine, 139
Arthritis pain, 133
Arthroses, 140
Autism, 11
Asai, Dr.Kazuhiko, 63
Ayurvedic, 119

B

Back pain, 143
Bacteria, 12, 18
BeneJoint, 80
Benzodiazepine, 110
Black cohosh, 123
Blood poisoning, 5
Blood pressure, 50
Blood-sugar levels, 6
Bone mass, 81, 84
Brain-damage, in children, 11
Brain power, 64, 97
Breast cancer, 41
Breast self-examinations, 43
Broccoli, 47
Bronchitis, 92
Burdock root, 123
Burgstiner, Dr., 69
Burns, 92

C

Calcium, 83
Calcium elenolate, 3, 147
Cancer, 10, 12, 19, 30, 39
Candida albicans, 9, 19, 21
Capsaicin, 80
Carbohydrate-binding proteins, 25
Cardiocysteine, 53
Cardiovascular disease, 61, 91
Cartilage regrowth, 77
CDC, 56
Chai-hu, 87
Chamomile, 124
Chapparal, 93
Chemotherapy, 25
Chinese medicine formulas, 35
Cholesterol, 6, 53, 104
Cholesterol levels, 55
Chondroitin, 78
Chronic fatigue syndrome, 15, 60
CHT, 36
Circulation, 6, 64
Combination hormone therapy, 36
Cold, common, 8
Coleus forskohlii, 115
Colostrum, 7
Cortisone-type drugs, 76
Cow's milk, 15
Crohn's disease, 20
Cryptosporidiosis, 11

Culturelle, 20
Cytokine, 9
Cytolog, 14

D

Damiana, 124
Dendranthema morifolium Tzvel, 37
Depression, 106, 107, 109, 125
Detoxification, 50, 64
Devil's apple plant, 29
DHA, 103
Diarrhea, 20
Diarrhea, in children, 14
Digestive disorders, 92
Disease, infectious, 3
DMARDs, 86
Docosahexaenoic acid, 103, 148

E

Eicosapentaoic acid, 104
Electromagnetic field, 142
Encephalitis, 4
Endocrine disrupters, 121
Energy, 65, 74, 125
Energy currents, 141
Entrainment, 51, 59
Epimedium grandiflorum, 119
Epstein-Barr virus, 4
Essential fatty acids, 104
Estrogen, 121, 125
Evista, 82
Exfoliant, 33

F

Farabloc, 139
Faraday, Micheal, 139
Fat burning, 125
FDA, 44, 56, 64, 82
Feverfew, 145
Fibromyalgia, 13, 15
Fish oil, 104
Fight or flight response, 60
Free radicals, 12, 50
Freeze-Frame, 59

G

Gan-cao, 87
Ganoderma lucidum, 37
Garlic, 5
Germanium, organic, 63
Ginger, 49, 145
Gingko biloba, 99, 124
Ginseng, 99, 119
Gleason's score, 36
Glucosamine-based products, 78
Glycoalkaloids, 29
Glycyrrhiza glabra, 37
Gonorrhea, 5
Gotu kola, 125
Grape-skin extract, 49
Green tea, 49
Growth hormones, 128
Gut flora, 18

H

Headache, 15, 60, 109, 143
Heart disease, 56, 57, 104, 129
Heart health, 6
Heart health support, 6
Heart Math, Institute of, 59
Hepatitis, 69
Herpes, 93
Herpes symptoms, relief from, 91
High blood pressure, 5, 60, 109
HIV, 4, 11
Homocysteine, 54, 57
Hormone levels, 121
Hormone refractory, 36
Hormone replacement therapy, 122
Huang-chin, 87
Hypertension, 59, 137

I

Immune booster, 21, 27, 74, 125, 129
Immune catalyst, 64
Immune dysfunction, 13
Immune system, 3, 8, 15, 16, 125,
Immune-system support, 16, 89
Impotence, 129
Infections, 74
Infections, surgical, 5
Infertility, 129
Inflammation, 12, 16, 125,
Influenza, 4
Infopepetides, 13
Inositol, 105

Index

Insomnia, 109, 112
Interferon, 65
Ipriflavone, 82
Isatis indigotica, 37

J

Joint pain, 15, 78, 142

K

Karposi's sarcoma, 95
Kavalactones, 110
Kava kava, 109
Kinia, Ivan M.D., 130
Klinik St. George, 13

L

Lactobacillus acidophilus, 19
Lactobacillus bulgaricus, 19
Lactobacillus G.G., 19
Lactoferrin, 7, 13
Lam, Herman, 112
Lane labs, 79
Larrea tridentata, 92
Larreastat, 91
LDL cholesterol, 6, 10, 48, 50
Leaky gut syndrome, 18
Libido, 123, 125
Limbic system, 112
Lung efficiency, 129

M

Magnesium citrate, 145
Malaria, 4
Male hormones, 39
Mammograms, 41
McCully, Kilmer, M.D., 53
Mediterranean Diet, 5
Memory, 102, 104
Meningitis, 4
Meningoencephalitis, 15
Menopause, 122
Menstrual cramps, 143
Menstrual problems, 143
Mental capacity, 60, 103
Mental function, 57, 104, 112
Metastasis, 7
Migraine, 143, 145, 146
Mobility, 84

Modified citrus pectin, 25
Mood swings 109
Mother's milk 7
Muira Puama 115
Muscle pain 13, 109
Muscle tone 129
Mulitple Sclerosis 69
Myalgias 13
Myalgic pain 16

N

National Institutes of Health (NIH) 41
Natural killer (NKCell) 12, 27
NDGA 94
Nervous system 61
Neural synapses 104
Neurotransmitters 102
Nonsteroidal anti-inflammatory drugs 75, 76
NSAIDs 75, 86, 135

O

Obsessive-compulsive disorder 105, 107
Ocular disturbance 9
Olive-leaf compound 3,
Olsen, Margaret M.D. 31
Omega-3 fish oil 148
Oral herpes 95
Osteoarthritis 76
Osteoporosis 83, 125
Oxygen enhancer 64, 65

P

Pain relief 65, 84, 112, 133
Panax pseudo ginseng 37
Panic attacks 107, 112
Panic disorder 105
Pantocrine 129
PC Spes 35
Penis 119
Phagocytosis 4
Phantom pain 140
Phenylalanine 136
Phosphatidylserine (PS) 99
Phytochemicals 47
Pneumonia 5

Polyphenols 48
Postsurgical pain 143
Prednisone 18
Premenstrual syndrome 122
Probiotics 17
Progesterone cream, natural 122
Progesterone therapy 122
Prostaglandins 129, 135
Prostate cancer 118
PSA levels 39
Prozac 106, 110
PSA test 36
Psoriasis 69
Pygeum africanum 117

R
RA Spes 85
Rabdosia rebescens 37
Red-date extract 102
Red deer antler velvet 127
Rheumatic pain 142
Rheumatism 92
Rheumatoid arthritis 76, 85, 89, 91, 92
Riboflavin supplements 145
Rosen, Allen MD 32

S
Saw palmetto, 37, 117, 124
Scuterllaria baicalensis, 37
Self-exams, 41
Sensor Pad, 42
Serotonin levels, 107 146
Shan-yao, 87
Shark Cartilage therapy, 75
Shingles, 15, 95
Shoulder pain, 141
Siberian ginseng, 123
Sinusitis, 5
Skin Answer, 30
Skin cancer 26, 29
Skin problems, 33
Sleep aids, 110
Sleeplessness 110
Smart bugs, 3
Snakebite, 92
Soy, 82

Spinal column syndrome, 141
Sports injury, 143
SSRIs, 107
Steroids, 77
Stinging nettle, 117
Stress, 112
Stroke, 10
Substance "P," 78
Superfoods, 47
Synovitis, 78
Synthetic hormones, 121

T
T cells, 14, 16, 125
Testicular cancer, 121
Testosterone, 115, 119
Tse-hsieh, 87
Thymic formula, 69
Thymic glandular tissues, 69
Titus County Memorial Hospital, 56
Tomato antioxidant, 49
Toothache, 109
Toxins, 65
Tuberculosis, 5
Tumeric, 49

U
Upjohn Pharmaceuticals, 5

V
Velvet, deer antler 127
Viagra 115, 116
Viruses, 92
Vision problems, 10
Vitamin B_6, 56, 145
Vitamin B_{12}, 56
V-Power, 115

W
Wild oat straw, 124
Wild yam cream 121
Willow bark, 145
Wu-chia-pi, 87
Wu-wei-zi, 87

X
Xp-100, 135

Y
Yee, Robert Dr., 88
Yen-hu-suo, 87

Z
Zorivax, 92

Health Sciences Institute

This book has been based on the research of the **Health Sciences Institute**. Our monthly newsletter is designed to give you private access to hidden cures, powerful discoveries, breakthrough treatments, and advances in modern, underground medicine.

Whether they come from a laboratory in Malaysia, a clinic in South America, or a university in Germany, our goal is to bring the treatment that work, directly to the people who need them. We alert our members to exciting medical breakthroughs, show them exactly where to go to learn more, and help them understand how they and their families can benefit from these powerful discoveries.

Members of the **Health Sciences Institute** have the opportunity to take advantage of special reports, incentives, and products. Subscribe now by calling the member services hotline at (410) 223-2611. Or just fill out the form below and return to:

Health Sciences Institute
Order Processing Center
P.O. Box 925
Frederick, Maryland 21705-9913

••

Membership Form

❏ **YES!** I would like a one-year subscription to the **Health Sciences Institute** newsletter for the low price of $49. (That's 12 confidential *Members Alerts!*)

Name: _____
Address: _____
City: _____
State/ZIP: _____
Phone Number: _____
(in case we have a question about your order)

❏ My check is enclosed for $ _____ made payable to the **Health Sciences Institute.** *(MD residents add 5% sales tax)*

❏ Please charge my: ❏ Visa   ❏ MasterCard   ❏ AMEX
Card no.: _____
Exp. Date: _____
Signature: _____

HSI-HSUC3

"My Prostate Problems Are Gone...Bless You"

Just released: the all-new, revised edition of *Miraculous Breakthroughs for Prostate and Impotency Problems*. This thorough healing guide for every man over 35 is now available to men who are concerned about their prostate—and to women who are concerned about their men.

Surgical procedures on the prostate are among the most commonly performed operations in America. With impotence and incontinence as common side effects, it's now wonder men fear prostate disease and surgery. This book defeats fear by telling all sides of the story and gives every man reason for the hope of return to vigor and vitality. It also tells you what doctors often don't—for many men, nature offers far better alternatives than surgery.

• For example, one patient decided to take the natural healer and tonic revealed in Chapter 3 before scheduled prostate surgery. Very shortly after beginning the healing doses, the man noticed his prostate troubles were gone. His urologist canceled the surgery!

• In another case, one patient named Bill had a prostate so swollen he visited the restroom every 20 minutes. Yet, in less than a month of the natural remedy on page 35, Bill's symptoms eased, and within two months, he was sleeping through the night again.

• Another patient, Larry R., was told his prostate would be surgically removed. He took two natural supplements revealed on page 36 and noticed improvement within 10 days. In a month, all signs of prostate problems had disappeared!

Even if your prostate is healthy, you should follow this natural way of male health as a preventative measure. The table on page 38 tells exactly what to take.

Father Hohmann, a priest, was diagnosed with terminal prostate cancer. His doctor considered his case hopeless and told the priest to make his peace and retire. But he wasn't ready to die. Using an herbalist's prescribed remedy given on page 59, Father Hohmann found a cure "nothing less [than a] miracle."

Have your prostate battles left you feeling hopeless? See page 60 for the most potent natural remedy of all, able to help even cases declared hopeless. This super-potent male remedy has helped bring relief to the toughest prostate complaints *without doctors, drugs, or surgery*! Not getting enough of the one essential mineral given on page 26 can lead to infertility, and, in severe cases, impotency.

Dr. Rudolph Sklenar, a German medical doctor, popularized the male potency elixir named on page 55 after he noticed the robust health of elderly Eastern European and Russian peasants. The men boasted of their lovemaking prowess well into their nineties.

"I'm not a health expert or any type of nutritional specialist; I am just an average guy—a guy who used to suffer from prostate disease. But thanks to William Fischer's latest book, I am no longer bothered by my prostate. I spent literally years searching for a doctor who could help me, but I found no relief. Finally, I gave up and resigned myself to living with the pain. My wife bought me a copy of *Miraculous Breakthroughs*, but I was sure it would be of no use. Boy, was I wrong!

"There is so much sound advice, I can't imagine any man not finding something that agrees with his body and his lifestyle. I was thrilled to discover that two products worked especially well for me. The answer to my problem was so simple." Mr. J.C.B., New York.

"Several years ago I developed some problems with my prostate gland. The troubles looked innocent enough at first, but they eventually grew and the situation got more serious. Someone loaned me a copy of the original edition [of the book].

"Well, before I knew it, my problems had eased up. My doctor was surely surprised (shocked would be a better word), and I made sure I checked with him every so often. My prostate problems are gone. I'm happier than I've ever been and believe it or not, I feel I have the energy of someone half my age! Bless you!" Mr. C.H., California.

The objective of the book is to help men prevent prostate problems and cancer. For those who are quietly suffering with these conditions, the goal is to find ways to relieve the pain, reverse the disease, and restore the body to vibrant natural health.

Miraculous Breakthroughs for Prostate and Impotency Problems is the owner's manual for the male body. You owe it to yourself and to your loved ones to read this book and discover the healing possibilities it offers.

Call Toll-Free Today! 1-888-821-3609

Or, send us this coupon along with your payment to the address below. Your copy of **Miraculous Breakthroughs for Prostate and Impotency Problems** will be packaged discreetly and delivered to your door.

❑ Please send me ____ copies of **Miraculous Breakthroughs for Prostate and Impotency Problems**.

Name:_____

Address:_____

City:_____State:_____ Zip:_____

Phone: (_____)_____
(In case we have a question about your order)

❑ I have enclosed my check or money order for $19.95 *plus* $4.00 shipping and handling for each copy.

❑ Charge my: ❑ VISA ❑ MasterCard ❑ AMEX

Card No:_____ Exp._____

Your Priority Code: PSUC3

This book comes with a *100% Satisfaction Guarantee*. If you are not fully satisfied, you may return it within one year for a complete refund. No questions asked.

Agora Health Books • P.O. Box 977 Dept. PSUC3 • Frederick, MD 21705-9838

Slow down aging with this Russian longevity formula

Fight cancer with this Italian wonder "drug" that has been featured in The New England Journal of Medicine

Eat fatty food (including red meat) and still lower your risk of heart disease using this proven German method

This Turkish salep will make your love life wild again

Natural Health Secrets from Around the World

More Than 1,600 Proven Remedies You Can Use at Home

As you read this, more than eight million people in Sweden are slashing their risk of heart disease by as much as 60%. Over one billion more in China and Japan are medically "bullet-proofing" their bodies against cancer. Countless others are getting rid of back pain, impotence, headaches, hair loss, and fatigue. And all without surgery or dangerous prescription medications. They are using the healing power of natural medicines and drugs that have been developed over thousands of years in countries all around the globe. For example:

• In India, **arthritis pain** is routinely eliminated with this "miracle" root. Add it to your diet and you too may begin to live pain-free...See page 113.

• This Chinese tea remedy really works for **menstrual cramps**. (And it's available in your local health food store.)...See page 364.

• People from Mexico, Saudi Arabia, Cambodia, and Burma use this versatile miracle treatment to treat **impotence, increase energy, boost stamina,** and **treat headaches**...See page 286.

Finally available in America

Until now information about alternative health remedies such as these was not publicized in America. And no wonder. The U.S. medical establishment is very uncomfortable with the fact that millions of people in all different parts of the world are living healthier, happier, and longer than most Americans—and without expensive and dangerous drugs and surgical procedures.

Dr. Glenn Geelhoed, an expert on international medicine, worked with a group of researchers to create a useful and practical guide that any American could use to take advantage of the preventative and curative traditions that other cultures have been using to keep themselves healthy for hundreds of years.

The result is the 650-page *Natural Health Secrets* volume, a book dedicated to the idea that there is so much you can do before your body fails—so much you can do to prevent disease and live longer—without high-tech, intrusive procedures. You can do so much today—right now—to rid your life of pain and recover the energy and vitality of your youth. And it's all within easy reach.

Safer and less expensive

The fact is, these natural healing methods are often safer and much less expensive than mass-market drugs. Time and again, natural remedies have proven effective where the conventional approaches have failed. And every one of these 1,600 remedies can be found or used at home. For example:

• Russians can drink all night and still **avoid hangovers**—their secret is surprisingly simple.

• Don't let **headaches** keep you from enjoying life...use the super-fast remedy discovered by North Africans—it may be the best treatment yet!

• Find out how Italians smoke, drink, and eat plenty of pasta...yet still have a lower incidence of **heart disease** than Americans.

• Check your kitchen cupboard—you might have this powerful American Indian aphrodisiac on hand to use whenever, however, and how often you wish.

• Look younger with this Caribbean remedy for **wrinkles**.

- Relieve **back pain** with an exotic fruit ointment popular with pain sufferers in the Fiji islands.
- Boost your **energy level** without caffeine or drugs—ancient Olympians used this safe, high-energy stimulant to improve stamina and performance.
- In the depths of the Burmese jungle people routinely live past 100—their secret not only guarantees **longevity** but keeps them **virile, energetic,** and **healthy** year after year.
- Add this Seminole Indian remedy to your diet and you may never come down with a **cold** again.
- This Russian treatment for **hemorrhoids** gives quick, long-lasting relief—yet it costs a fraction of the price of commercial preparations.

In recent years, the public has been clamoring for more information and access to natural remedies from overseas. American medical institutions are now researching many of these natural methods and medicines. The results verify that many natural remedies do have substantial scientific validity. For example:

- A report in *Annals of Internal Medicine* concludes that garlic, a Chinese doctor's staple, lowers **cholesterol**.
- Some scientists believe that bark from this 100-year-old European tree contains a chemical compound that might provide an effective treatment for **cancer**.
- A Harvard Medical School team reported that an extract from this southern "weed" helps treat **alcoholism**.
- A **natural sex stimulant** used by men in West Africa for centuries has been tested for effectiveness at Stanford Medical School—and the results are very encouraging!

Why is Natural Health Secrets so different?

To tell the truth, I don't believe there's another resource anywhere that reveals so many useful alternative natural remedies. Other health references—even those published by America's top health publishers—tend to focus on Western medicine and American approaches to health and healing. There's nothing wrong with this except that these offer a very limited perspective. There's a whole world of natural remedies and treatments available to you. Why shouldn't you know about them?

I have no doubt this book will show you secrets that could make your life—and the lives of people you love—healthier, happier, longer. *Natural Health Secrets* may very well be the most useful resource for natural medicines available today. And for a limited time, you can own your copy today for just $29.95.

For The *Fastest* Service Use Your Credit Card And Call Toll-FREE

1-888-821-3609

❏ **YES!** I want the wisdom and invaluable healing secrets of cultures around the world! Plus, I have nothing to lose by ordering now. With your **365-day Money-Back No-Risk Guarantee,** I get a *full year* to use *Natural Health Secrets* on my own…and if I'm not *completely and utterly satisfied*, all I have to do is return it for a total refund of my purchase price! That's a great deal. So please send me *Natural Health Secrets* today for just $29.95 + $5.00 shipping and handling (Total: $34.95). Here is my address and how I wish to pay:

Name:_____

Address:_____

City:_____ State:_____ Zip:_____

Phone: (_____)_____
        (in case we have a question about your order)

Your Priority Code: **NHUC3**

❏ Please charge my: ❏ Visa ❏ MasterCard ❏ American Express

❏ Enclosed is my Check or Money Order made payable to Agora Health Books.
(Maryland residents add 5% sales tax)

Card #:_____ Expires:_____

Agora Health Books • PO Box 977 Dept. NHUC3 • Frederick, MD 21705-9838

Black Listed Cancer Treatment Could Save Your Life

Six-time Nobel Award Nominee Discovers Two Nutrient Cancer Breakthrough

A top European cancer research scientist, Dr. Johanna Budwig, has discovered a totally natural formula that not only protects against the development of cancer but has actually helped people all over the world who had been diagnosed with incurable cancer and sent home to die.

After three decades of research, Dr. Budwig, a six-time nominee for the Nobel Award, found that the blood of seriously ill cancer patients was invariably deficient in certain important substances, including phosphatides and lipoproteins. Without these, cancer cells grow wild and out of control. Blood analysis also showed a strange greenish-yellow substance instead of the healthy, red, oxygen-carrying hemoglobin that should be there, explaining why cancer patients become weak and anemic. This startling discovery led Dr. Budwig to test her theory.

She found that tumors gradually receded when these natural ingredients were replaced over a three-month period. The strange, greenish-yellow elements in the blood were replaced with healthy red blood cells as the phosphatides and lipoproteins almost miraculously reappeared. Weakness, anemia, cancer symptoms, and liver dysfunction disappeared, and vitality was restored.

Dr. Budwig then discovered an all-natural way for people to replace these essential substances their bodies so desperately needed. By simply eating a combination of just two natural and delicious foods, cancer was not only prevented but in case after case was actually succesfully treated.

After more than ten years of solid clinical application, Dr. Budwig's natural formula has proven successful where many orthodox remedies have failed. Dr. Budwig's formula is now used therapeutically in Europe for the prevention of: cancer, arteriosclerosis, stroke, cardiac infraction, stomach ulcer, prostate disorder, arthritis, eczema, aging, and immune-deficiency syndromes.

Here's what Dr. Budwig's followers say:

Magda W. was told by an expert doctor that the cancerous tumor causing swelling under her eye would have to be cut out, because the malignancy was too far advanced for radiation treatment. "I was afraid for my life, but being a young woman, couldn't bear the thought of such disfigurement. When I heard about Dr. Budwig's natural formula, I was skeptical but desperate for help."

Afterwards, the doctors at the university hospital gave her many exhausting tests, and one even told her, "If I didn't have your previous x-rays and medical history in front of me, I wouldn't believe you ever had cancer." Magda says, "I never thought using Dr. Budwig's formula would be so successful. My whole family and I are very grateful."

Scotty A. experienced blurred vision, loss of balance and coordination, and a complete shutdown of his bladder. He went to a nearby medical research center for a series of tests, which showed arachnoidal bleeding due to a brain tumor. Scotty was sent home from the hospital to die in peace.

A friend hurried to his bedside with hope in the form of Dr. Budwig's formula. "After eight weeks on the diet, I was able to walk unaided for the first time in months. My health improved so rapidly that I was soon able to return to my work part time. The Budwig diet saved my life!"

You will learn all about Dr. Budwig's formula and other surprising facts that can save your life in the new edition of the book *How to Fight Cancer and Win*. For example:

• A popular method of cooking steak is equivalent to the harm done by smoking 600 cigarettes in a row. A simple change in cooking that you can make completely neutralizes this harmful effect. See page 70.

• Japanese people have a very low incidence of **colon cancer**. See why on page 56.

• See page 58 for the amazing nutrients that **stopped tumors** in tests at Albert Einstein College of Medicine.

• Did you know that, contrary to popular belief, eating the right amount of butter, eggs, milk, cheese, and well-marbled beef can actually **lower harmful cholesterol levels**? See page 67.

• This little-known, little-eaten food is a powerful cancer fighter. The National Cancer Institute published the results of a study that determined this food contains an active anti-cancer element with the power to slow the development of mammary tumors. Documented healing and disease-fighting effects of this nutrient include **treatment of aging, digestive upsets, prostate disease, sore throats, acne, fatigue, sexual problems, allergies**, and a host of other problems. See page 156.

• This vegetable may have preventive and even curative powers over cancer and is considered the first line of defense against cancer. See page 191.

• According to the National Cancer Institute, adding just 200 micrograms daily of this natural substance found in our soil might prevent cancer. Experts now say that cancer rates across the board could be cut as much as 70% if the general population took this small amount daily. Japanese women who do have just one-fifth the rate of **breast cancer** of American women who don't. Learn what natural food contains this important substance on page 252.

You will find the answers to all of this and much, much more in *How to Fight Cancer and Win*. At the turn of the century, cancer claimed the life of one person in thirty. Today cancer kills one in five.

"Your book and the work of Dr. Budwig is truly great! I know of a woman in my church who had a brain tumor and became blind. After taking Dr. Budwig's formula, her sight came back! I met her mother just the other day—she told me her daughter is now free of cancer! Thank you." Ruth K.

"*How to Fight Cancer and Win* is a milestone in publishing history. I have never read a more down-to-earth, practical resume of cancer prevention and treatment. It's one of the most important books every written on cancer and degenerative disease." Edward Steichen, M.D.

Call Toll-Free Today! 1-888-821-3609

Or, send us this coupon along with your payment to the address below. Your copy of *How to Fight Cancer and Win* will be delivered to your door.

❑ Please send me ____ copies of *How to Fight Cancer and Win*.

Name:_____

Address:_____

City:_____ State:_____ Zip:_____

Phone (_____) _____
(In case we have a question about your order)

❑ I have enclosed my check or money order for $19.95 plus $4.00 shipping and handling for each copy. *(Make payable to Agora Health Books. MD residents please add 5% sales tax.)*

❑ Charge my: ❑ VISA   ❑ MasterCard   ❑ AMEX

Card No:_____

Exp._____

Signature:_____

This book comes with a *100% Satisfaction Guarantee*. If not fully satisfied, you may return it within one year for a complete refund, less shipping and handling. No questions asked.

Agora Health Books • P.O. Box 977 Dept FCUC3 • Frederick, MD 21705-9838

Manuscript Of Ancient Chinese Healing Techniques Reveals
How to Breathe Disease Out of Your Body
Secret Methods Date Back Over Four Thousand Years—Harness the Most Fundamental Life Force Known to Eastern Disciplines

We recently discovered an obscure, paper-bound manuscript that turned out to be the only known record of a secret system of Chinese healing. It's a system of breathing techniques combined with simple body postures, handed down for centuries by traditional Chinese doctors. These powerful techniques use the principle of chi, considered by Eastern disciplines to be the energy source that carries life through your body.

• Imagine successfully **treating cancer, colds, viruses, ulcers, heart disease, arthritis, impotence,** and discomforts from **menopause**—simply by breathing...

• Imagine banishing **headaches, fatigue, nervousness, stiffness** and **pain**, simply by breathing...

• And imagine harnessing the most powerful force in your body, channeling it, and using it to heal yourself...

• Imagine all this, and you will understand how important a discovery we've made.

The techniques are based on a force called *chi*. (Also known as "ki," or "qi" by Eastern philosophies.) It's the same force the ancient Vedics of India called "prana," and was identified as "pneuma" by the classical Greeks.

Chi is the vital, essential force behind all life. One ancient saying states that "Chi is the mother of blood." Acupuncture, traditional Chinese medicine, shiatsu and reiki are all based on the principles of chi, and work on the paths through the body that this energy flows through.

In fact, anyone familiar with Eastern forms of exercise and meditation has probably heard of chi. Tai chi, yoga, qi gong, karate, and Zen meditation all teach correct breathing as the basic necessity for practice. That's because correct breathing focuses the power of chi, and radiates it through your body.

Here are just a few of the techniques you can use to heal and prevent disease:

• Treat **cancer** with "ton-ren-mai-zan." (In this technique, you'll also learn to use two secret pressure points, known as dan-chun and hya-kkai, along with the breathing. These are critical areas where chi can be stalled in the body, causing illness and disease.)

• Relieve **angina** with "fei-je-jan-yo"—simple movements that Western doctors may not discover for another hundred years...

• End **fatigue** with "pei-ta-chuen-shen." (This technique uses a secret system of tapping and patting the body—more concentrated than massage, but more gentle than acupressure—to free energy throughout the body. It's fast, it's easy, and the results are amazing.)

• Banish **arthritis** pain with "woo-rong-tan-jao." Forget drugs! They simply mask pain and suppress inflammation. Healing techniques such as woo-rong-tan-jao combine gentle movements, breathing, and the body's own energy to relieve and heal afflicted areas.

• Successfully treat **asthma** with "chu-chi-jun-pi." This technique will remind you of the most classic yoga postures. Simple and easy—but combined with a certain stretch and proper breathing, the lower lungs are expanded and used. At the same TIME, healing energy is freed throughout your chest, lungs, and entire body.

• Boost your **sex** drive with "jo-tie-nho-hao." Western medicine keeps looking for a magic pill to boost your sex drive and cure impotence. Unfortunately, it's usually just another drug—with side effects and long-term damage that's only discovered way down the line. But this technique uses a simple principle and gentle internal movements to stimulate your body's natural functions. It's absolutely the simplest and safest way in the world to rejuvenate yourself.

• Find deep, restful **sleep** with "an-chi-wan-jo" (once again, using secret pressure points can produce miraculous results in the body...)

Each one of these techniques is beautifully diagrammed and carefully explained. They're easy to follow, and easy to do. No confusion, no misunderstanding. The author has brought these ancient secrets alive, and delivered them right into your hands. And, in *Healing with Ki-Kou: The Secrets of Ancient Chinese Breathing Techniques*, you'll find over 125 pages of these ancient secrets, covering almost every imaginable pain and illness.

For The *Fastest* Service Use Your Credit Card And Call Toll-FREE
1-888-821-3609

❑ **YES!** I want to learn how to heal myself with breathing. Plus, I have nothing to lose by ordering now. With your **60-day Money-Back No-Risk Guarantee**, I get two months to use *Ki-Kou: The Secrets of Ancient Chinese Breathing Techniques* on my own…and if I'm not *completely and utterly satisfied*, all I have to do is return it for a total refund of my purchase price! That's a great deal. So please send me *Ki-Kou: The Secrets of Ancient Chinese Breathing Techniques* today for just $24.95 + $5.00 shipping and handling (Total: $29.95). Here is my address and how I wish to pay:

Name:_____

Address:_____

City:_____ State:_____ Zip:_____

Phone: (_____)_____
  (in case we have a question about your order)

❑ Please charge my: ❑ Visa ❑ MasterCard ❑ American Express

❑ Enclosed is my Check or Money Order made payable to Agora Health Books.
  (Maryland residents add 5% sales tax)

Card #:_____ Expires:_____

Agora Health Books • PO Box 977 Dept. CBUC3 • Frederick, MD 21705-9838

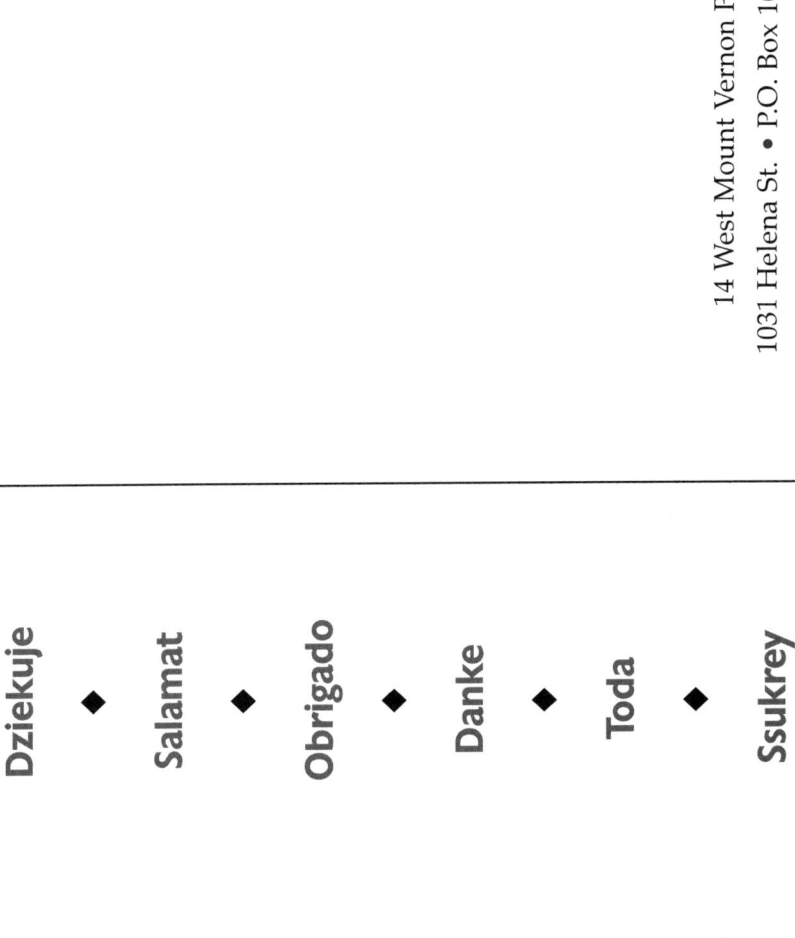

Bill Bonner
Owner and Founding Publisher

14 West Mount Vernon Place • Baltimore, MD 21201 • USA
1031 Helena St. • P.O. Box 1051 • Fort Erie, ON L2A 6C7 • Canada
U.S. Customer Service • Telephone: (1-410) 783-8440 • Fax: (1-410) 230-1258
Email: agoraintl@agora-inc.com

Dziekuje

◆

Salamat

◆

Obrigado

◆

Danke

◆

Toda

◆

Ssukrey

Agora International
INCORPORATED

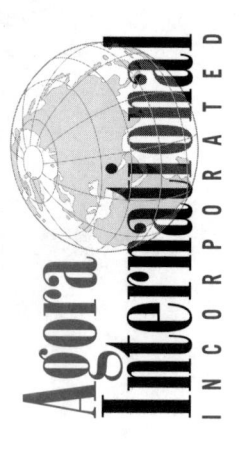

Thank you for your recent order of an Agora International, Inc. product.

We are always striving to bring you the most up to date and time-sensitive information available. As always, please let us know if we can be of any assistance.

Sincerely Yours,

Thank You
- **Merci**
- **Gracias**
- **Grazie**
- **Arigato**
- **Aciu**